The Lose Your Belly Diet
Change Your Gut, Change Your Life

by Travis Stork, M.D.

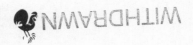

WITHDRAWN

BANTAM PRESS

LONDON • TORONTO • SYDNEY • AUCKLAND • JOHANNESBURG

TRANSWORLD PUBLISHERS
61–63 Uxbridge Road, London W5 5SA
www.penguin.co.uk

Transworld is part of the Penguin Random House group of companies
whose addresses can be found at global.penguinrandomhouse.com

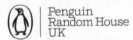

First published in the United States of America in 2016 by Ghost Mountain Books, Inc.

First published in Great Britain in 2017 by Bantam Press
an imprint of Transworld Publishers

A CIP catalogue record for this book
is available from the British Library.

ISBN 9780593079317

Typeset in 11/16pt Arno Pro
Printed and bound by Clays Ltd, Bungay, Suffolk.

Interior Design and Production: Dovetail Publishing Services,
www.dovetailpublishingservices.com

Penguin Random House is committed to a sustainable
future for our business, our readers and our planet. This book
is made from Forest Stewardship Council® certified paper.

61325

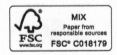

MIX
Paper from
responsible sources
FSC® C018179

1 3 5 7 9 10 8 6 4 2

Dedication

It may seem silly, but I'm dedicating this book to my pup of nearly 17 years, Nala. She was a rescue whom I adopted during my first year of medical school. I wasn't planning on getting a dog but it was pet adoption day while I was at the store. As she cowered in the corner with her fur coat covered in red clay, she kept looking my way. After a few minutes, I knew she was going home with me. Since that time, she's been by my side. From every exam in medical school to the writing of this book, she has taken every step with me. Even if her steps these days are taken a bit more slowly!

Note to Readers

The anecdotes in this book are used to illustrate common issues and problems that I have encountered and do not necessarily portray specific people or situations. No real names have been used.

As with all books, this one contains opinions and ideas of the author. It is intended to provide helpful and informative material on the subjects addressed in the publication. It is sold with the understanding that the author and publisher are not engaged in rendering medical, health, psychological, or any other kind of personal professional services or therapy in the book. The reader should consult his or her medical, health, psychological, or other competent professional before adopting any of the concepts in this book or drawing inferences from it. The content of this book, by its very nature, is general, whereas each reader's situation is unique. Therefore, as with all books of this nature, the purpose is to provide general information rather than address individual situations, which books by their very nature cannot do.

The author and publisher specifically disclaim all responsibility for any liability, loss, or risk, personal or otherwise, which is incurred as a consequence, directly or indirectly, of the use and application of any of the contents of this book.

Acknowledgements

I want to personally thank Alice Lesch Kelly for her dedication to this book and her excitement for helping me bring this important project to life. A special thanks to Lisa Clark: your guidance and commitment to getting things right is refreshing and quite frankly awesome. Andrea McKinnon for helping me hatch this idea while waiting at the airport in Austin, TX. And to everyone else who played a role in the development and evolution of this book, I thank you!

Contents

INTRODUCTION

Your Gut Health/
Weight Loss Opportunity

Let me start by saying that I love food. Let me also say that the most important health lesson I've ever learned is to let food be my medicine and not my poison. This has been my guiding principle for quite some time now. But here's the truth: our knowledge of *how* food affects our health and weight is always changing and evolving. *The Lose Your Belly Diet* is a book I was inspired to write because of our rapidly changing knowledge of the human gut microbiome and its effect on our health and weight. If you don't know what "human gut microbiome" means, don't worry, because you soon will! It's exciting stuff, and my goal is to be there with you every step of the way as you learn how to optimize gut health *and* maximize weight loss—especially the loss of harmful belly fat.

This plan focuses on food choices and portion control strategies that help you eat more of the high-quality foods that nourish you and make you feel full and satisfied, and fewer of the low-quality foods that lead to excess weight gain and fat accumulation. It checks *all* of the healthy-eating boxes while filling you up with delicious, enjoyable foods.

The Lose Your Belly Diet is an evolution of *The Doctor's Diet*, a book I wrote a couple of years ago. I loved that book, because it's such an effective, easy-to-follow plan and was the way I used to eat. But since that book came out, we've learned so much important new information about gut health and the impact of beneficial bacteria on our overall health and weight. It's changed the way I eat and it should change the way you eat, too.

This plan tells you the how and why of enjoying life-supporting foods, and it does so without deprivation. In fact, it gives you more freedom and flexibility than pretty much any diet out there. Not only does it encourage you to eat an abundance of gut-supporting foods, but it makes room for bread, pasta, and other whole grains that so many diets cut out these days.

And even more fantastic: this diet makes room for things like chocolate, wine, and coffee, which not only make life worth living (in my humble opinion) but appear to be beneficial for your gut bacteria, too!

A Boom of New Information

I wanted to write this book because I believe we're in the midst of a dramatic change in our understanding of human health. The discoveries that scientists are making about the human microbiome are so important that I feel we should *all* start implementing them into our lives immediately.

Here's where it all started. I keep a pretty close eye on medical news. Not only is it my job—both as a physician and as the host of *The Doctors*—but it's also my personal passion. I want to live the longest, healthiest, most vibrant life possible, so I'm always on the lookout for ways to improve my health and the health of my family, friends, patients, and viewers.

During the past few years, one of the areas that has grabbed my attention on an almost daily basis is the growing field of human microbiome research—the study of the various tiny organisms that live in our bodies, especially in our bellies. Nearly every day, another piece of research reveals previously unknown connections between our overall health and the well-being of the microbes that live in our gut.

This may come as a surprise. We're accustomed to thinking of bacteria and other microbes as being bad—and some, such as E. coli or salmonella in contaminated food, can indeed cause serious illness. But these bacteria bullies give their fellow microbes a bad rep. Most of the bacteria and other microbes in our bodies are actually very good; they do amazing things, such as working with our immune system to fight off dangerous invaders and helping our intestines digest food. When the microbe communities in our guts are healthy—when they are diverse and in balance—there seems to be a higher likelihood that we will be healthy, too. And, when our personal microbe community is in bad shape, it raises some big red flags for our overall health. Having an unhealthy personal microbiome has been linked to problems with immunity, gastrointestinal health, and autoimmune diseases such as rheumatoid arthritis, allergies, and asthma. There's also evidence that it may be associated with obesity and other difficult-to-solve health problems.

This is a time of great discovery for microbiome researchers. In fact, the findings about gut microbes have been so promising that I am convinced the human microbiome is one of the most exciting new frontiers in medical discovery that we've seen in quite some time.

Buddies in Your Belly

In a nutshell, here's what we know about the human microbiome: When scientists analyze individual people's microbe communities, they find that healthy people have many more beneficial microbes overall and a much greater variety of microbe species in their bodies than less-healthy people. We don't know all the details yet—hundreds of microbiome studies are still under way—but one thing is clear: having a vibrant, balanced, diverse microbe community is the way to go. So it makes really solid sense for us all to be protecting and supporting the population of our personal microbiome.

Gut microbes play such a crucial role in our health that it's kind of amazing that it's taken so long for us to start giving them the attention they deserve—but better late than never. Now that we are learning about how to take care of our gut microbes, it's time to start figuring out how to incorporate that research into our everyday life choices.

That's exactly what we'll do in *The Lose Your Belly Diet.*

The Lose Your Belly Diet is built around a simple concept that comes up over and over in human microbiome research: making choices that protect and support the microbes in our guts paves the way for better health—not just for our guts, but for our whole self. These choices do more than just help sustain our gut microbes. They lower our odds of developing various diseases. And they raise our chances of reaching and maintaining a healthy weight, and of burning off dangerous belly fat. In the pages that follow, I'll tell you how to do all that and explain the many ways—most of which are fairly simple—that you can immediately start to protect and support the microbes in *your* gut.

I like to think of the microbes in my belly as my Little Buddies who are helping me stay healthy every day. I owe my Little Buddies a lot, and I want to do everything possible to take care of them.

Your Personal Gut Guide

Despite my enthusiasm for the subject of gut health, I understand that not everyone wants to delve into the down-and-dirty details of it the way I do. I get it: most people don't relish the idea of reading the latest *JAMA* study on faecal microbiota as they drink their morning coffee. (Yes, I admit, I've done this.) But living a long, healthy, vibrant life is a major goal for just about everyone I know. So, even if you don't like thinking about stool samples, you probably do like the idea of finding out simple ways that you can apply the cutting-edge discoveries about microbiome health to your everyday life.

That's where *The Lose Your Belly Diet* comes in. I'm not a gut researcher, but I am intensely interested in microbiome research. The patients I work with and the people I talk to every day want to know what they can do to improve their health, boost the quality of their life, feel better, and live longer. So think of me as your own personal gut guide. I've digested the major microbiome studies (I know, bad pun) with one goal in mind: to figure out how you and I can apply this new information to our daily lives and diets.

The recommendations in *The Lose Your Belly Diet* reflect the latest research about gut health. But here's something important to keep in mind. Although we have learned so much lately, there are still many things we don't know about gut bacteria and how best to support it. So when we come across questions that don't yet have clear answers—for example, the jury is still out about the benefits of probiotic supplements for the general public—I promise to be frank with you. When we don't know whether A is better than B or C, I'll level with you and share whatever guidance is available to help you make choices that are best for you.

But don't think too much about what we *don't* know, because there is so much we *do* know about how to support your Little Buddies. Using the advice in this book, you can start taking steps to help your gut bacteria immediately.

Fuelling Your Little Buddies

Many of my microbiome-enhancing recommendations in *The Lose Your Belly Diet* involve food, because the foods we choose to eat and avoid have a major impact on the health of our Little Buddies. Because diet plays such a huge role in microbiome health as well as overall health, I've created a diet plan that supports your gut and your entire body—a plan that does a super job of feeding your gut and enhancing your overall health while helping you slim down (if that's your goal).

But this book is way more than just a diet. *The Lose Your Belly Diet* will provide you with all kinds of recommendations that reflect the growing knowledge we have about a healthy gut microbiome. I'll walk you through all the changes you can make—from the foods you buy and the medicines you take, to the way you think about dirt and germs. I'll also cover some of the choices you make as a parent that will positively benefit your family's microbes.

Most of these changes are easy to make. For example, the Little Buddies in your gut benefit when you eat raw or less well-cooked foods, so I'll share some delicious ideas for including more raw produce in your diet, including a new kind of veggie dish that is an innovative twist on an old American favourite. Some remarkably simple changes help, too: believe it or not, simply cooking your wholegrain pasta to the al dente texture that most chefs prefer—rather than boiling it until it's very soft—can give your gut microbes a boost because it leaves more of the fibre in the pasta intact, which makes a better feast for your gut bacteria.

To make things even easier for you, I've developed simple meal plans and quick, delicious recipes that will make it a breeze for you to follow *The Lose Your Belly Diet* for the rest of your life. And I'll show you, step-by-step, how you can start eating some of the foods that are especially helpful for gut health, such as fermented foods and probiotic foods that deliver beneficial bacteria to your gut.

Full-Body Benefits

A nice side effect is that when you do good things for your gut, you do good things for your physique, too. *The Lose Your Belly Diet* can be customized to support your own personal weight goals, whether you want to take off excess pounds or just look leaner. You'll find that by following *The Lose Your Belly Diet*, you'll not only control your weight, but you'll also be making choices that lower the risk of potential killers such as heart disease, diabetes, and certain kinds of cancer. That's pretty great news.

Here's one more exciting benefit you can expect when you start following *The Lose Your Belly Diet*. Our focus is on the inside of your body, where as many as a thousand different kinds of microbes are playing a part in your everyday health. *The Lose Your Belly Diet* can help you shed the harmful belly fat that interferes not only with your health, but with the way you look in your swimsuit. While you nurture your gut with *The Lose Your Belly Diet*, you'll also be supporting just about every other part of your body.

About This Book

In *The Lose Your Belly Diet*, I start off by sharing information with you about your gut microbes and the various things that help them. Then I get down to brass tacks, giving you specific advice on diet and other lifestyle choices that protect, support, and increase gut bacteria. If you're anxious to get started on *The Lose Your Belly Diet*, feel free to jump ahead and get going right away—it starts on page 133.

The Lose Your Belly Diet is so simple that you can easily start following it at your next meal. You probably already have many of the recommended foods in your refrigerator or pantry.

If you do decide to fast-forward to *The Lose Your Belly Diet*, make sure to come back and read these beginning chapters when you have a chance. I've found that it's much easier to make smart choices about diet and health when you have a clear appreciation of why those decisions make sense. I don't want you to opt for an apple over a bag of crisps only because it's what I told you to do. I want you to embrace *The Lose Your Belly Diet* because it's what *you* want and because *you* are making an informed choice based on your knowledge and commitment to your Little Buddies and yourself. When you really understand the "why" of good health as well as the "how to," you're much more likely to stay motivated and reach your goals.

So feel free to jump ahead to *The Lose Your Belly Diet* if you're excited to start making changes. But don't forget to learn all about why it's so good for you and your Little Buddies!

I'm happy to tell you that change happens fast when you start following *The Lose Your Belly Diet*. In one study, researchers found that improvements in microbe diversity—one measurement of gut health—began to occur surprisingly quickly among study participants who started making microbiome-supportive diet changes. Researchers thought it might take weeks, months, or even years for improvements to occur, but much to their surprise, gut health started getting better within *days* of making simple diet adjustments. To me, that's a sign that our bodies want to be healthy, and they are primed and ready to receive our help and to start benefitting from positive change right away.

With all that in mind, let's get going—there's no time to waste! Your Little Buddies are ready for you to rock their gastrointestinal world!

PART

I

What's Going On in Your Belly?

When you were a kid, you probably spent a fair amount of time rooting around in your garden. And you probably discovered that there are a lot more living things in a garden than most of us realize. At first glance you might have seen a squirrel or a couple of birds. But when you lifted up a big stone, a whole new world would come into view—an entire community with all kinds of bugs and worms and little tiny critters with lots and lots of legs.

That's kind of what it's like in our bellies. Check out your belly in a mirror and you don't see much aside from skin and a belly button. But if you could peek inside, a whole new world would come into view—solid organs, blood vessels, nerves, and yards and yards of intestines.

Then, if you were to delve even deeper—and if you could strap on some kind of high-tech sci-fi glasses with super-microscopic vision—you'd see an even more amazing world, a community that is bursting with life. You'd see the microbes that make up your own personal slice of the human microbiome.

In this section of *The Lose Your Belly Diet*, we're going to focus on what's going on in your belly—what kinds of microbes live there, what jobs they do, and the roles they play in disease and weight gain. We'll also start looking at some of the steps you can begin taking—starting today—to repair damage to your gut. By making some simple changes, you can go a long way toward protecting and supporting the Little Buddies in your belly.

CHAPTER

1

Meet the Microbes

You think of yourself as an individual, but in reality, you have a huge number of Little Buddies riding around in your gut.

Your belly is populated by somewhere in the neighbourhood of about 100 trillion microbes. Wow! I don't know about you, but I find it pretty hard to wrap my head around that number, which is a 1 followed by 14 zeroes. Although your gut microbes' numbers are enormous, their footprint is small: all together they weigh a total of just two to six pounds. The microbes in your gut have a huge number of cells—10 times more than all of the other cells in your body. And they contain a total of about 1,000 more genes than are present in every other part of your body. Amazing!

Even if you can't quite picture all those organisms nestling in your belly, it does make sense for you to know about them—and to thank your lucky stars that you have them. In fact, we humans wouldn't be able to survive without them.

This community of microbes—which scientists refer to as the human microbiome—helps us in many ways, some of which we understand and many of which we have yet to discover. But like every other community of living things, gut microbes do their jobs most effectively when they are residing in an environment that supports and protects them. In that respect, our Little Buddies are no different than most living beings, including you and me.

I'd like to tell you a little about these microbes, because understanding a few things about them will help you do a better job of taking care of them. Don't worry, I'm not going to give you a medical school lecture on the gut—just a quick intro to the incredible population of microbes in your belly.

Gut Superstars

Microbes are tiny organisms that are so small they can be seen only with a microscope. Most of the microbes in your body are bacteria, but there are also viruses, fungi, and several other kinds of microbes in and on you. Healthy adults are home to up to 1,000 different species of bacteria. All of the microbes in the human body together are referred to as the human microbiome; I refer to the microbes in your own body as your personal microbiome. Most of these microbes live in your large intestine, but they're also found throughout your digestive system (which also includes your mouth, oesophagus, stomach, small intestine, rectum, and anus) and on your skin, genitals, nose, ears, and sinuses. Since most microbes are bacteria and the vast majority of them are in your gut, they're frequently referred to as "gut bacteria."

Human microbe communities are a little like our fingerprints: no two are alike. Although certain species of bacteria are found in most people's guts, some are unique. Bacteria vary from person to person, from family to family, and from population to population. Families tend to have similar microbiome profiles—probably because of genetic factors and because families live in close proximity to one another and eat similar foods. We even share some of the same gut bacteria with our pets.

Personal microbiomes also differ based on geography. The microbiome profile of an American's gut is likely to be different from a Brazilian's or a South African's, for example—and a New Yorker's would probably be different from a Texan's. Many factors contribute to this, including genetics, hygiene, diet, health history, previous infections, antibiotic exposure, environmental toxins, and more. As humans have evolved, so too have the microbes in our bodies—and as you'll soon see, not always in a good way.

When we talk about having a healthy microbiome, we're referring to two main considerations: the *total number* of beneficial Little Buddies in our bodies, and the number of *different species* of microbes that call our bodies home. A

A Sequence of Events

You may be wondering why the human microbiome is getting so much attention lately—I mentioned earlier that hardly a day goes by that I don't read a new study about the human microbiome. But why is all that news coming out now?

Amazingly, the human microbiome was not generally recognized until the late 1990s. It wasn't even mentioned when I went to medical school. But a lot has happened since then. Most of the discoveries about the human microbiome have been spurred by big progress during the last decade or so in the field of gene sequencing. This is a process that allows us to identify genes based on the specific makeup of their DNA. Gene sequencing was first used to identify human genes. However, after researchers started decoding the human genome, they realized that in order to understand the human body completely, they'd also need to understand and sort out the genetic makeup of the microbes that live within it. So they turned their focus to the human microbiome. As gene sequencing identified, decoded, and catalogued the genetic makeup of gut microbes, scientists began using this information to launch in-depth studies about how the various kinds of microbes affect overall health.

The National Institutes of Health Human Microbiome Project (HMP), which was established in 2008, has supported much of the research that explores connections between health, disease, and the condition of the human microbiome. If you're interested in delving more deeply than this book does into the nuts and bolts of the microbiome, a great place to start is the HMP website (www.hmpdacc.org).

healthy microbiome is diverse, which means it has a greater number of species of microbes. When scientists analyze the gut microbiomes of people who are not healthy, they often find fewer species of microbes than they find in the guts of healthier people. Although there is some question as to whether lack of diversity leads to disease or vice versa, scientists feel confident that microbiome diversity is a very positive thing, and lack of diversity isn't good.

How do all of these microbes enter our bodies? It starts at birth (or possibly before birth—scientists aren't completely sure). As babies move through the birth canal during delivery, they are exposed to the microbes in their mothers' vagina. This is referred to as "colonization." More microbes enter their bodies during breast-feeding and as they interact with people and their environment, and it continues throughout life. Our personal microbe communities reach maximum diversity during adolescence, and if we treat them well, they can stay relatively stable until our senior years.

Keeping Our Little Buddies Healthy

As we make our way through life, various things—good and bad—can impact the health of our Little Buddies. I'll tell you more about all of these things throughout the book, but here's a quick rundown.

Based on what we know so far, the microbes in your gut community benefit from a healthy diet; exposure to people, animals, and plants that carry a diverse mix of microbes; being born via vaginal delivery; and being fed with breast milk during infancy. There's even evidence that exercise helps our Little Buddies, too.

Eating a healthy diet is one of the best ways that we can support our gut bacteria. That means choosing more of the foods that help our Little Buddies thrive—especially the dietary fibre found in fruits, vegetables, whole grains, nuts, seeds, and pulses—and choosing fewer refined foods, sugars, processed meats, and other foods that we know are not very good for our health and that seem to be detrimental to our gut microbes, too. In particular, when we don't feed our gut bacteria the high-fibre food they need, they can starve, die off, or be overtaken by less beneficial bacteria. Or they may feed on the mucus membranes that line our intestines (a bit of an unpleasant thought, if you ask me), which can lead to inflammation and other health problems.

Some of the other things that can harm our gut microbes include chemical cleaning products, certain health conditions, antibiotic medications, antibiotics used in our food supply, delivery via Caesarean section, formula feeding, and alcohol abuse. We'll look at all of these more closely in upcoming chapters.

Those are some of the things we know so far, but I'm sure there are many more discoveries on the horizon. For example, studies in mice have found that cigarette smoke damages their gut microbes—no surprise there, since cigarette smoke has been found to cause harm to so many other parts of the body. These results come from mice studies, but I'll bet you 100 to 1 that the same will be found with people. I'm also guessing that as this type of research progresses, we'll discover that many of the other types of environmental toxins that damage cells and organs—air pollution, pesticides, heavy metals, you name it—may hurt our gut bacteria. And I think we may also find that many of the factors that boost our health in other ways—good sleep and stress relief, for example—may turn out to benefit our Little Buddies as well. In this respect, I think we have a lot in common with our little friends.

Our Changing Microbiome

It's kind of ironic: just as we are discovering the amazing contribution that our gut microbes make to our health, we're also realizing that over the past few generations, the human microbiome has been changing, especially in developed countries such as the United States. The typical Western lifestyle seems to be fairly harmful to our Little Buddies. "Our microbiome has changed significantly over the past century, and especially over the past 50 years," said New York University microbiologist Martin Blaser in an article in *The Atlantic* magazine. "We're losing microbes with each generation; they are going extinct. These changes have consequences."

Among the consequences Blaser is referring to are dramatically increasing rates of allergic diseases such as asthma, eczema, food allergies, and some other health problems that are much more common today than they were in past decades. This is no surprise to me—I'm someone who has suffered from asthma and seasonal allergies for much of my life, and since I've been focusing much more on eating to feed my gut microbes, my symptoms have improved significantly. Coincidence? Maybe, but it certainly isn't hurting that I'm decreasing my body's overall inflammation with the changes I've made in my diet and lifestyle.

Unfortunately in modern society we eat too much of the foods that act like poison to our health and our Little Buddies: highly processed foods and "natural" foods raised in an unnatural way with synthetic pesticides and antibiotics. We also eat too few of the foods that act like medicine for our health and Little Buddies: fibre-rich vegetables, fruits, whole grains, pulses, nuts, and seeds, for example. Also playing a role in the destruction of our Little Buddies' health is the rampant overuse of antibiotics (more on this later because it upsets me that healthcare providers are largely to blame for this!) and changes in the ways in which babies are often delivered (more C-sections) and fed (formula rather than breast milk).

Scientists also point to the cleanliness of our world in the twenty-first century. By relying so heavily on antimicrobial sanitizers and other germ killers, we also reduce our exposure to the good Little Buddies that help build up a healthy microbiome.

So what can we do about all this? Some of it is beyond our control, but fortunately there are many steps we can take to improve the health of our microbiome community and subsequently our overall health. With *The Lose Your Belly Diet*, we'll focus on the changes that are within our control.

The Choices We Make

Before we go any further, I want to stop for a minute and talk about something important. A few of the things I mentioned that can harm the microbiome might upset you. Maybe you gave birth by C-section, ate a poor diet for many years, were prescribed a lot of antibiotics, or smoked cigarettes. If so, I hope you'll think about it this way: What's done is done. When it comes to your health, it's not helpful to spend a lot of time looking back and regretting past decisions. Instead, focus on now. For instance, I was formula fed. But I don't spend a second of my life worrying about that, and I certainly don't blame my mum. You can't change the past—but the future is wide open. What matters is what you do now, beginning this very moment. Let go of any regret you may have and use that energy to start making choices *today* that will benefit your health and start rebuilding your gut microbiome from this day forward.

Coming Up

Now that you've met your microbes, we'll take a look at why it's so important to have a healthy microbiome. In the next chapter, we'll talk about some of the many jobs your Little Buddies do every day.

CHAPTER
2

Your Very Busy Buddies

The Little Buddies in our guts perform so many important jobs that many scientists think of the human microbiome as a "forgotten human organ" that is as important to our health as our heart, lungs, or liver. I like to picture all those trillions of microbes as busy workers in a teeming factory, where everyone is busy doing work that benefits our health.

We've known for a long time that gut bacteria exist in our bodies, but it's really only recently that we have figured out how many jobs they do. Take digestion, for example. We always assumed that the major players in our digestive system—the stomach, intestines, liver, gallbladder, and pancreas—did the lion's share of the job of breaking down our food to release and absorb nutrients and energy that can be used by the body. But now, on further study, we realize that our gut microbes also play a huge role in digesting food. It's kind of amazing— like thinking that instead of having five or six guys painting your house, there are actually 100 trillion.

When I first started immersing myself in my own education about the human microbiome, I discovered that the more I learned about how crucial gut microbes are to our health, the more I wanted to take care of my own Little Buddies. I think you'll feel the same way, so let's spend a little time doing a rundown of some of the ways they help us stay alive. Again, we won't go deep into the science, but a quick look should go a long way toward inspiring you to take the health of your gut microbes pretty darn seriously. I know I do.

Digesting your food. As I mentioned, your gut microbes help break down your food so your body can use it. Here's what that means: When you bite into a food—let's say an apple with peanut butter—digestion starts right away as your teeth grind it up and the juices in your saliva start to break it down. After you swallow, the mashed-up apple-nut mixture travels through your oesophagus to your stomach, where stomach acid and enzymes break down large molecules into smaller molecules that are easier for your body to absorb. Then, the apple-nut mush moves into your small intestine, where more digestive juices join the party and break down protein, fat, carbohydrates, and various nutrients so that they can be absorbed into your bloodstream to be transported throughout your body. What's left—fibre, mostly—travels through your large intestine, and anything that doesn't get absorbed leaves your body in the form of stool.

At every step of that process, gut bacteria are also busy working to break down that apple with peanut butter so your body can use it. To start with, your gut bacteria help manufacture some of those juices that start digesting food the minute you put it in your mouth. Gut microbes assist with the building of some of the enzymes, amino acids, and other chemicals that your body needs to digest food. They also work with your body to extract energy and nutrients from food. In fact, some foods, such as certain heavy-duty kinds of dietary fibre, are actually digested by our gut bacteria on our behalf.

When gut bacteria are out of whack—a condition that scientists refer to as "dysbiosis"—your digestive system may suffer. We believe that's true because people with digestive diseases tend to have fewer overall gut microbes and a smaller number of microbe species than healthy people. What's more, when your gut microbes are out of balance, your body may have trouble absorbing certain nutrients, which can lead to nutrient deficiencies, diarrhoea, wind, and various other unpleasant symptoms. The risk for certain diseases goes up, too.

Making vitamins. Most of the vitamins we need come to us through food. But several vitamins that we know of—vitamin B12, thiamine, riboflavin, and vitamin K, and perhaps some we don't yet know about—seem to be manufactured by gut bacteria in addition to coming to us through food. The belief is that bacteria need these vitamins, so they make certain types on their own using raw materials in our bodies—and what they don't need is released so that our bodies can use it. This is typical of the symbiotic relationship (symbiotic means that it's beneficial to both sides) between people and their gut microbes. Our Little Buddies help us by assisting with various important jobs, and we help them by eating meals and snacks. The food we eat feeds our gut bacteria, and they count on us to send down a new round of grub every couple of hours. This singular concept is something I've always believed: eating food should be viewed as a good thing, and the fact we are feeding our Little Buddies is part of the reason why.

Fighting "bad" bacteria. We've been talking about the good microbes in your body, but there are some not-so-good ones as well. For example, E. coli is a large group of bacteria found in foods, the environment, and the intestines of animals and people. Not all types of E. coli are bad, but a few can cause serious illness and even death. When your Little Buddies are in great shape, they can help you fight off dangerous types of E. coli before they make you sick.

Working with your immune system. Our immune system's job is to fight off dangerous germs (pathogens) that can harm us. But how does your immune system know when to attack and when not to? Lots of factors are involved in this very complex system, and one of them seems to be the gut bacteria. Scientists believe that a kind of communication goes on between your gut microbes and your immune system, and that your gut bacteria actually help "train" your immune system from an early age to know when to do battle and when not to. But when your gut bacteria are out of balance, this communication can be interrupted, leading your immune system to under-respond (allowing pathogens to cause trouble) or over-respond (causing your body to fight off good guys in addition to bad guys).

An over-responsive immune system causes a lot of potential problems. It can contribute to autoimmune diseases such as rheumatoid arthritis, coeliac disease, lupus, and a common type of hypothyroidism, to name just a few.

With autoimmune diseases, the body attacks healthy tissues as if they were invasive pathogens.

This is important, because various health problems are linked to immune dysfunction, including autoimmune diseases. We can't say that having a damaged gut microbiome causes these diseases, but in countries in which gut bacteria diversity has decreased over the past few decades—such as the United States—the incidence of many autoimmune diseases has increased.

Gut bacteria may influence the immune system in another way, too. When gut bacteria are out of kilter, you're at greater risk of inflammation in the lining of your gut. When the gut becomes inflamed, bacteria and other substances are more likely to be able to pass in and out of your gut—a situation referred to as "leaky gut." When the gut is leaky, things that should stay inside your gut can leak out, and vice versa, triggering an immune system reaction. Having leaky gut can cause your immune system to overreact in a way that not only harms your gut but could contribute to other diseases as well.

It really is starting to look like shortages and overgrowths of certain gut microbes make certain diseases more likely to occur. In that case, you may be wondering whether it's possible to transplant "good" microbes into people with health problems. If so, I like the way you think. Although it sounds like science fiction, the truth is, it's already starting to happen.

Little Buddies to Go

Forward-thinking medical researchers are trying an inventive new approach to helping people with damaged guts: they're taking some of the bacteria from healthy people and transplanting them to sick people. It's a process called "faecal microbiota transplantation," or FMT, and although it's still considered an experimental therapy, it's showing great promise for certain health problems.

One such problem is *Clostridium difficile* infection (CDI). CDI causes about half a million infections and at least 29,000 deaths in the United States each year; it is most likely to strike older adults, people in hospitals and nursing homes, people with suppressed immune systems, and people who receive medical care for conditions such as HIV, cancer, organ transplants, or inflammatory bowel disease. CDI can cause watery diarrhoea, fever, nausea, loss of

Should You Have Your Microbes Analyzed?

Several companies offer microbe analysis for people who would like to know more about what's going on in their gut. Is it worth it to have your stool tested?

My answer for the majority of folks is, not yet. Microbe testing can be expensive and is not ready for prime time. We simply don't know enough about microbe counts to be able to understand definitively what various results mean. And the only real advice to give people who get poor results is to eat more probiotics and fibre, avoid unnecessary antibiotics, and do all of the other things we're covering in this book—which all of us should be doing anyway, no matter what our gut analysis might find.

In the interest of science, I had my stool tested. But the results didn't really change anything for me. These really are the early days of microbiome research, and testing has a long way to go. Someday I'm sure that microbe testing will be cheaper and we'll better understand what to do with the results. In the meantime, if you want to get tested like I did, there is certainly no harm in it. But you're better off spending that money on the healthy foods that we'll be discussing in this book.

appetite, and belly pain. It's hard to cure, and it often comes back over and over—a really nasty, annoying infection. Believe me, you don't want CDI.

Early studies with FMT show that it helps some CDI patients by restoring bacterial balance in their guts. To do the transplants, faeces samples are collected from healthy donors and are inserted into capsules. In one study, 20 patients with CDI received 15 FMT capsules on two consecutive days. Of the 20 patients in the study, diarrhoea and other CDI symptoms disappeared in 18—a 90 percent success rate, which is pretty fantastic for a condition that can be very hard to cure. Some of them saw their symptoms improve after just one FMT capsule.

Doctors are excited about the idea of treating CDI with FMT. (I know, lots of acronyms.) Ordinarily CDI is treated with antibiotics, but some strains are antibiotic-resistant, which means that none of our antibiotics can kill them. Having another treatment option for CDI could save lives, improve quality of life, and possibly help prevent the spread of antibiotic-resistant bacteria.

In the future, FMT may be used to treat other kinds of health problems, such as irritable bowel syndrome and Crohn's disease. It may even help with obesity—more about that in the next chapter. For now it's an experimental treatment. And it does have certain challenges. For example, not all FMT trials have had identical results—for reasons that researchers don't fully understand, sometimes FMT works well for CDI, and sometimes it doesn't. Also, we need to be sure that when we transplant faecal bacteria, we're not implanting harmful bacteria from donors. And there's the "yuck factor" as well—we are talking about taking other people's stool into our bodies, after all. But my guess is that these challenges will be overcome and you'll be hearing a lot about FMT in the future, not just for disease treatment and prevention but possibly to help address the obesity epidemic as well. The research is exciting, but please don't start swapping stool samples with your best friend!

Coming Up

Now you know a few of the ways that gut microbes work hard to help keep you healthy. In the next chapter, we'll look at how your Little Buddies may be influencing your weight—and your ability to burn off excess pounds.

CHAPTER
3

Microbiome Balance and Weight Gain

You've heard the statistics: 36 percent of adults in the United States are obese. An additional 33 percent are overweight. Only 31 percent of American adults are considered normal weight or underweight. The situation isn't much better for young people: about one-third of children and adolescents are overweight or obese. There's no way around it—too many of us carry more weight and fat than we should. And since excess weight is associated with a long list of health risks, we would be far better off if we could slim down.

We tend to blame America's weight problem on calories, framing it with a basic calculation of calories in versus calories out. When we eat too many calories and burn too few, we gain weight. And when we cut calories and step up our workouts, we lose weight. That's just basic mathematics, right?

Hold your horses. While it is true that eating more calories than you burn on a regular basis can lead to weight gain, and that cutting calories can help you lose pounds in the short term, the reality of the weight gain/weight loss equation isn't quite as simplistic as it sounds. Researchers are finding that other factors beyond just the arithmetic of calories consumed play a major role in weight. For example, personal metabolism—the rate at which each of us uses and stores energy from food—comes into the equation, too. Because of genetics, physiology, and a bunch of other considerations, your body probably burns and holds on to energy at a different rate than your best friend's body.

Even if you both were to eat exactly the same food and do precisely the same amount of exercise, you'd probably gain or lose weight at a different rate than your friend.

Additionally, researchers are now discovering that gut bacteria also seem to play a role in the complex process of weight loss and weight gain. We don't know exactly how much impact our Little Buddies have on our weight, but we're learning enough to believe that understanding the connection more fully may help us as we confront the obesity epidemic in the United States—and in our own bodies.

Just Getting Started

Don't get too excited—we don't have a silver bullet yet. So far, there are no gut bacteria pills or other breakthroughs that will magically melt off your extra weight or provide an overnight solution to the American weight crisis. But research into gut bacteria and weight has shown enough promise that it's definitely worthwhile for anyone with a weight problem to get serious about protecting, supporting, and increasing beneficial gut bacteria.

Cutting back on food calories and boosting exercise burn will always be a crucial part of successful weight management. But I believe that taking microbe-supporting steps like the ones I recommend in this book can make weight loss via diet and exercise more achievable and maintainable. And in the future, gut researchers might even figure out ways to develop bacteria-based treatments that could help tackle obesity in an even more direct way.

Looking for Links

Researchers have found a bunch of different connections between weight and gut bacteria. None of them paints a complete picture of how our microbiome might influence our weight, and vice versa, but they do sketch out some interesting possibilities.

Let's start with gut bacteria diversity, which is the variety of different species of bacteria in the gut. As I mentioned earlier, healthy adults tend to have a greater diversity of beneficial bacteria species in their guts than less-healthy adults. It also seems that lean people have more gut diversity than obese people. Think of the gut as a box of crayons: in lean people, you'd see every colour of the rainbow, and in obese people, you might see just a small number of reds, blues, and greens.

This doesn't mean that having a lack of diversity in gut bacteria *causes* obesity. It's also possible that gaining excess weight puts extra strain on our gut bacteria, or that the kind of diet associated with obesity doesn't adequately nourish them. But it does suggest a new area of research for scientists who are scratching their heads about the causes of the obesity epidemic. And in my opinion, it may help explain why losing weight is so very much harder for some people than for others.

Here's where we are right now. Studies have found that certain *types* of bacteria are more commonly found in the guts of lean people than in obese people. For example, researchers comparing the microbes in the guts of more than 1,000 volunteers found that having an abundance of a type of gut bacteria known as *Christensenellaceae* is linked with being lean, and having less is associated with obesity. More research is needed, of course, but it does suggest the possibility that having (or not having) certain bacterial strains or species could contribute to obesity. And it also suggests that certain bacteria may offer protection from obesity.

Why would some bacteria be linked with leanness, and others with fatness? There are a few possible reasons. Scientists have noticed that some microbes seem to be better at releasing energy and fat from foods than others—let's call them Fat Little Guys. If this is the case, then people with more Fat Little Guys would absorb more calories from their food and would gain more weight from the same amount of food than people with few or no Fat Little Guys. That might help explain why people who eat similar amounts of food gain different amounts of weight—for example, why you seem to gain weight even when you're on a diet, and your slender friend who eats cookies and ice cream non-stop never seems to gain an ounce.

There's more. Other research has found that in addition to more species of bacteria, lean people have as much as 70 percent more gut bacteria *overall* than overweight people. And countries with more overweight people tend to have less bacterial diversity in their guts. So, while we might not necessarily understand all the details of exactly how gut bacteria impacts weight gain or loss, I'm convinced that there's a link.

Other Connections

The Little Buddies in your gut may also affect weight in these ways:

How hungry you feel. Gut bacteria may influence the action of ghrelin, leptin, and other hunger and satiety hormones. Because of this, it's possible that the presence (or absence) of some kinds of bacteria could contribute to your feeling hungrier than you actually are, and you may not get the message as clearly as you should when you've eaten enough to satisfy your physical hunger. We often blame overweight or obese people for not having the willpower to eat less. But if gut bacteria are influencing the action of hunger hormones, we would understand that much more than willpower is at play.

How hot you burn. We know that gut bacteria play an important role in immune function. And it's likely that they influence the amount of inflammation in our bodies. When your immune system isn't working well, levels of inflammation throughout your body can rise. Out-of-control inflammation can lead to the storage of excess belly fat and can make weight loss more difficult. It can also damage healthy cells, tissues, and organs, such as the heart and the brain. It can make your cells less responsive to insulin and thus interfere with blood sugar levels. It can also damage healthy cells, tissues, and organs, such as the heart and the brain, and can contribute to the growth of tumour cells.

Chronic inflammation—which is inflammation that continues over long periods of time—has been linked to a wide range of diseases, including heart disease, cancer, metabolic syndrome, diabetes, Alzheimer's, arthritis, type 2 diabetes, and stroke. Although genetics and some other factors affect chronic inflammation, it seems that a damaged gut microbiome contributes to the condition as well.

How you store fat. Gut bacteria are heavily involved in digestion, and it's likely that they help out with the regulation of insulin and blood sugar, as well as the process of storing fat for future use. Just as there are species of bacteria that are linked with leanness and obesity, I'm guessing there probably are species that specialize in efficient fat storage, too. As we tease out the details of how gut bacteria specifically influence fat storage, we will likely be able to develop specific treatments to help our bodies to store less fat, especially in our bellies. The good news is that I'm confident you can begin using food at this very moment to start to improve your gut bacteria, and this book will show you how.

Transplanting Bacteria

If it does turn out that some bacteria are linked to leanness and some to obesity, you might be wondering whether those Lean Little Buddies can spread the love a little. Wouldn't it be great if those of us who struggle with our weight could get a dose of bugs from some of those naturally slim people we all envy so much?

That might just happen someday. Remember the lean *Christensenellaceae* bacteria I mentioned? When researchers transplanted them into mice, the mice that received them were less likely to become overweight or obese than those that didn't receive transplants.

Some other studies with mice have had similar results. In one set of studies, researchers worked with identical twin mice that were bred to have no gut bacteria of their own. The researchers populated the guts of some of the mice with bacteria from lean humans, and some of the mice with bacteria from obese humans. Then they fed the mice identical diets. What happened to the mice is absolutely fascinating: those with gut bacteria from lean humans stayed lean, and those with bacteria from obese humans became obese. In these mice, the kind of bacteria in their guts seems to have determined whether or not they became obese.

There's more. When researchers added gut bacteria from the lean mice to the guts of the mice that had become obese because their guts had been populated with bacteria from obese humans, the mice that otherwise would have gained excess weight stayed lean. When the Lean Little Buddies faced off against the Fat Little Guys, the lean team appears to have won. This is very exciting stuff!

We don't know whether this will translate from mice to humans. But the results are promising. If the gut bacteria found in lean people seems to help them stay lean, perhaps we could transfer lean bacteria to overweight people. After all, as you may remember from chapter 2, faecal microbiota transplant, or FMT, has shown promise in helping people with the difficult-to-cure *Clostridium difficile* infection, or CDI. Can the same process be applied to weight managment? It's hard to tell just yet. Humans are a lot more complicated than mice, and it may take a while before this kind of research moves from laboratories and research hospitals to your doctor's office—or perhaps even your local pharmacy.

The hope is that someday, we'll be able to add Lean Little Buddies to supplements or food. Perhaps if we knew that bacteria X, Y, and Z helped with weight loss, we might be able to add them to probiotic foods such as yogurt, kefir, or a daily probiotic supplement. But we're not there yet, and we may not be for a while.

What You Can Do Now

In the meantime, there's plenty you can start doing right away, such as eating a wide variety of high-fibre foods. We know that *most* gut bacteria love high-fibre foods. Notice I say "most." Research suggests that the foods we associate with a poor diet—processed foods, refined foods, sugar, fatty meats, and so on—may actually be the go-to favourite fuel for Fat Little Guys that are linked with obesity. We don't know all the details, but it does appear that some kinds of obesity-linked bacteria flourish in people who eat a junky diet. And when these Fat Little Guys prosper, they may start to crowd out some of the Lean Little Buddies in the gut.

I realize this all has something of a cops-and-robbers feel to it. I fully admit that I am simplifying some very complex research with metaphors that make a complicated topic easier to understand. But I want you to get the idea behind it all: When we eat junky foods, we may be giving aid to the enemy. When you don't feed your Little Buddies enough of the high-fibre food they need, bad things may happen to them. They may not have the vitality they need to stand up to obesity-linked bacteria. Or, they may starve and die off. Or, they may feed on the mucus membranes inside your intestines, which could damage your intestinal walls and contribute to inflammation. But, when we eat high-fibre foods like those recommended in this book, we are giving the Lean Little Buddies the fuel that best allows them to help us.

While the researchers continue to figure out some of the specifics over the next few years, you and I can start making changes right away. Put this book down, grab an apple, take a bite, and you'll be giving your Lean Little Buddies the help they need to do their jobs.

I've often said that food is our best medicine—and it can also be the best medicine for our Little Buddies.

Coming Up

Obesity isn't the only health problem that is linked to the diversity of gut microbes. Lots of other conditions have connections to gut health, too. In the next chapter we'll look at how our personal microbe communities may be influencing our health—and the ways in which positive change can benefit our bellies.

CHAPTER

4

Better Gut Health, Less Disease

As an emergency room doctor, I see countless people debilitated by chronic disease—emphysema patients barely able to breathe, heart attack victims doubled over with terrifying chest pain, stroke victims struggling to speak. The hardest part for me as a doctor, though, is knowing that so many of these diseases could have been prevented if these patients had made different choices. Heart disease, stroke, obesity, type 2 diabetes, and lung cancer are not only the most common diseases in America, but they're also the most preventable.

On the flip side, however, I also see an enormous number of people who are living happy, healthy, energized lives because of the lifestyle choices they make every day. I know that it's not always easy to practise good health habits. But if you spent a day in the ER with me, you'd see how worthwhile it is to take care of your body and your health.

We've known for a while that making a few really important choices—quitting smoking, improving your diet, exercising regularly, and limiting alcohol intake—can significantly lower your risk of developing chronic diseases. Now, we may be adding another recommendation to that list: taking care of your gut microbes.

Although we still have a lot to learn about connections between gut microbes and chronic disease, scientists are finding some dramatic links between microbial imbalance and health. And they're discovering that taking care of our Little Buddies is an important way to safeguard ourselves from disease. Let's take a look at how these connections might affect you.

The Big Three

Three of the major chronic health conditions in the United States are cancer, heart disease, and type 2 diabetes. Together these three diseases kill about 1.3 million Americans every year. Not every case of heart disease, diabetes, or cancer is caused by lifestyle choices, but many are. And we know changing the way we live can significantly lower our risks of developing these diseases. One of those changes seems to be taking better care of our gut microbes.

Take cancer, for example. Various studies are uncovering fascinating links between gut bacteria and cancer. For example, one study found that having a particular type of gut bacteria raised the risk of developing stomach cancer. Another found connections between colorectal cancer and imbalances in certain specific types of gut bacteria. And in animal studies, researchers have found that mice with some strains of gut bacteria were more likely than other mice to develop lymphoma or more likely to experience DNA damage that leads to lymphoma.

Does that mean that gut bacteria imbalances cause cancer? I wouldn't go that far. But it does suggest that if we can find ways to balance the microbes in our guts, we may be able to reduce cancer risk.

Imbalances in gut microbes seem to affect heart disease risk as well. We know that red-flag problems with gut bacteria trigger inflammation—and we know that inflammation raises the risk of heart disease. So it's no surprise that research is beginning to find links between poor gut microbe diversity and heart disease. For example, one study found that an imbalance of microbes in the gut is associated with a higher risk of heart failure. Other research hints at the possibility that the presence of certain bacteria in your gut can impact your heart's sensitivity to factors such as high LDL ("bad") cholesterol. This is an area of research that's in its infancy, but researchers hope that as they learn more about heart disease and gut bacteria, they'll be able to develop microbiome-based therapies to treat people who have already developed heart disease.

As for type 2 diabetes, which affects about 10 percent of Americans, research suggests that having specific microbes in the gut may offer protection.

Banking Bacteria

Unfortunately, certain cancer treatments may not be so great for your Little Buddies. Cancer is frequently treated with chemotherapy, which uses one or more very strong drugs designed to disable or kill cancer cells. Chemo drugs can be highly toxic to all living cells, which is why people who get chemo often experience severe nausea, diarrhoea, hair loss, and other side effects.

Well, it looks like chemo harms gut microbes, too. One study found that chemotherapy caused a "profound disruption of the intestinal microbiome," which is probably not at all surprising to anyone who's undergone this gruelling cancer treatment. But here's something to think about: researchers are looking at the possibility of having patients "bank" their gut bacteria—store some of their stool, that is—before chemotherapy treatment so that their Little Buddies can be implanted back into their guts after treatment. I love the idea of cancer patients being able to hold on to their Buddies and reintroduce them to their guts after their treatment ends!

In chapter 3, we talked about the fact that certain types of bacteria are more commonly found in the guts of lean people than in obese people. That also seems to be true when researchers compare the bacteria in people with and without type 2 diabetes.

It's possible that some bacteria are better than others at supporting the action of insulin in the body. And it's possible that in the future, we may be able to improve insulin sensitivity by transplanting gut bacteria from healthy volunteers into the guts of people with diabetes. But in the meantime, more research is needed before we can leap to the conclusion that microbe transplants will be a new treatment for diabetes. For now, the best strategy for reducing type 2 diabetes risk—and keeping the disease in control if you already have it—is to live a healthy lifestyle and lose excess weight.

Other Health Conditions

As gut researchers explore the connections between microbial imbalance and various kinds of disease, they often start out by noticing something very basic: When the beneficial microbe populations in a person's gut are healthy—when they are strong, diverse, and present in great numbers—that person is more likely to be healthy. And when the microbe populations in a person's gut are out of balance and lack diversity, the person is less likely to be healthy.

Take irritable bowel syndrome (IBS), for example. IBS is a gastrointestinal condition that affects 10 to 15 percent of adults in the United States. People with IBS can experience a range of symptoms, including abdominal pain and changes in bowel movement patterns (diarrhoea and/or constipation). Researchers have found that people with IBS have less gut microbe diversity than healthy people without IBS. What's more, people with IBS have smaller numbers of bacteroidetes, a type of gut bacteria.

Bacterial imbalances have also been found in people with inflammatory bowel disease, or IBD, which affects more than a million Americans. In people with IBD, the immune system attacks the cells of the intestines and produces chronic inflammation. Although the two most common types of IBD, Crohn's disease and ulcerative colitis, have genetic components, researchers have found that microbe imbalances in the gut also play a part in the development of IBD. It may be that in a person with a genetic predisposition to IBD, the genes related to the disease are more likely to "turn on" when their gut microbes are out of balance. And since gut bacteria influence the immune system and the body's inflammatory response, it's not surprising that problems with gut microbes could raise the risk of this inflammatory disease.

Another set of conditions linked to gut microbes are those related to allergies. During the past few decades, the incidence of allergic diseases has gone up dramatically. For example, since 1997, the rate of food allergies in children went up by 50 percent, and the prevalence of skin allergies in kids shot up by 70 percent. Researchers believe that these increases in allergies are probably due in part to imbalances in kids' gut microbes, which can be caused by an increase in the use of antibiotics in children, reduction in kids' exposure to beneficial bacteria in the environment, and other factors that have a negative impact on their Little Buddies.

There also appears to be a link between imbalanced gut bacteria and a variety of other health conditions, including rheumatoid arthritis, diabetes, multiple

What Happens When You Eat a Gut Bomb?

We've all eaten gut bombs—those big, heavy meals that leave us groaning with unhappiness. Loaded with grease, calories, salt, and sugar, gut bombs don't just make you feel bad—they do a job on your gut, too.

Think back to the last time you ate a gut bomb. Maybe it was a huge bacon burger and a gigantic side of fries with soda. Or maybe it was a big plate of greasy fried chicken surrounded by a mountain of potato salad, coleslaw, and baked beans. Whatever it was, think for a minute about how it made you feel: sluggish, heavy, bloated, and exhausted, no doubt. It may even have caused symptoms such as wind, intestinal cramping, and even constipation or diarrhoea.

Eating a gut bomb doesn't just weigh down your gut; it actually triggers the release of brain chemicals that have a negative impact on your mood.

One of the wonderful things you can look forward to on *The Lose Your Belly Diet* is that after eating a meal, you'll feel 180 degrees different than you do after ingesting a gut bomb. Instead of feeling like you swallowed a two-ton truck, you'll feel light, healthy, and ready to take on the world, rather than wanting to disappear into the couch. Your mood will be better and your gut will be happier. Sounds pretty good to me!

sclerosis, cardiovascular disease, *Clostridium difficile* infection (again, an infection that causes diarrhoea and other intestinal ailments), mental health problems such as anxiety and depression, and possibly even autism. Although we don't know exactly how having a healthy gut microbiome might reduce the risk of each of these conditions, researchers are anxious to figure it out, because understanding it could lead to new treatment options.

When it comes to research into the ways in which our microbes influence our risk of chronic disease, these are still early days. But the good news is that the lifestyle changes that help our gut microbes have already been shown to lower the risk of many diseases. You don't need to know the exact mechanisms involved. Just start making the healthy lifestyle changes in this book and you'll immediately begin lowering your risk of chronic disease.

Coming Up

There's no doubt about it: good health and a vibrant microbiome go hand in hand. But how quickly can you start to improve your gut environment? You'll have to read the next chapter to find out. But I'll give you a hint: when I found out the answer to that question, I couldn't stop smiling.

CHAPTER
5

Start Repairing Gut Damage TODAY

Okay, we've covered a lot of territory so far. You understand what your gut microbes do, why they're so important to your health, and the impact they may have on your weight and your risk of disease. Now it's time to start looking at the changes you can make to start repairing gut damage and supporting your Little Buddies.

Our twenty-first century environment contains loads of things that harm our gut microbes, including antibiotics in our foods and drugs, environmental toxins, and foods that harm rather than help our bodies. More on that later. But for now, the good news is that we can take significant steps to repair our damaged guts—and those changes can start making a difference sooner than you may think.

I believe that the most important step you can take to protect and support your Little Buddies is to start eating more dietary fibre. We know this for sure: a low-fibre diet simply doesn't provide your Little Buddies with the food they need. One study after another has found that switching to a high-fibre diet can give gut bacteria a big boost. The rest of your body benefits, too. Giant piles of research have shown that people who eat adequate fibre have a lower risk of various chronic health conditions, such as heart disease, obesity, diabetes, some kinds of cancer—you name it.

It all comes down to this: eating the kinds of foods recommended in *The Lose Your Belly Diet* is simply one of the best things you can do for your gut and your entire body.

Fast-Track Changes

So we know that dietary changes matter. The question is, how quickly can diet changes help you and your Little Buddies? You may think it takes weeks or months or even years. But it's actually much quicker than that, according to gut researchers.

To figure out exactly how fast diet changes could impact the bacteria profile in people's guts, Duke University researcher Lawrence A. David and his colleagues conducted a fascinating study. The researchers knew that previous research in mice had shown that the animals' personal microbiome could be altered quickly. For these laboratory mice, switching from a high-fat, high-sugar "Western" diet (like the diet eaten by so many Americans) to a lower-fat, higher-fibre diet resulted in changes to the animals' gut microbes within just one day. One single day! But would the same be true for humans? David and his colleagues didn't know, so they set out to see what they could learn about human responses to diet changes.

The researchers prepared two diets. The first was a high-fibre, plant-based diet that included lots of fruits, vegetables, pulses, and grains. This diet included cereal for breakfast, fruit for snacks, and vegetables, grains, and pulses for lunch and dinner.

The second diet was an animal-based diet composed of meats, cheeses, and eggs, and virtually no dietary fibre. This diet included bacon and eggs for breakfast, pork and beef for lunch, cured meats and cheeses for dinner, and snacks of pork rinds, cheese, and salami. Both of these diets, which contained equal numbers of calories, are obviously extreme, but the researchers hoped that by using diametrically different diets, clear results would be produced.

Once the diets were designed, it was time to test them on human volunteers. Researchers recruited six men and four women between the ages of 21 and 33—a small number of volunteers, for sure, but enough to get the ball rolling. For the first four days of the study, the volunteers ate their usual diets. Then for five days, they followed either the animal-based diet or the plant-based diet designed by the researchers. After those five days, the volunteers took a break from study foods and ate their usual diets for a few days—a step that's referred to as a "washout period" because it allows volunteers' bodies to return to their pre-study states. Then for five days, volunteers ate the study diet that was the opposite of the first.

Throughout the study, the scientists analyzed the study subjects' faeces—proof that being a microbiome researcher isn't necessarily a glamorous job!

The researchers were pretty impressed when they tallied their results.

Drumroll, Please

Analysis showed that both of the diets—the really high-fibre diet and the fibre-free diet—each began having an impact on the volunteers' gut bacteria within three or four days. Not only did the scientists see changes in the abundance of bacteria in the high-fibre group, but they also saw changes in genetic activity in some of the bacteria in the volunteers' guts. And they found that volunteers who ate the fibre-free diet had higher levels of a type of bacteria that is associated with the development of inflammatory bowel disease.

"These results demonstrate that the gut microbiome can rapidly respond to altered diet," the researchers wrote when they published their results.

"We found that the bacteria that lives in people's guts is surprisingly responsive to change in diet," says David, assistant professor at the former Duke Institute for Genome Sciences and Policy and one of the study's authors. The changes that researchers thought might take weeks, months, or years started to happen in just days.

I was totally on the bandwagon about following a microbiome-supporting diet before I read that study. But after I read it, my commitment was complete. I couldn't wait to start eating foods that would protect, support, and increase my gut bacteria. My guess is that you feel that way right now, too. That's why our next step takes a look at exactly which kinds of food will help your Little Buddies thrive.

Coming Up

Pull a chair up to your kitchen table. Tie a napkin around your neck. Grab a knife and fork. It's time to start eating. In the next section, we'll look at all of the fantastic foods that you can begin eating today to feed your Little Buddies and start boosting your gut health right away.

PART
II

Foods That Feed Your Gut

When we doctors receive our degrees, we take a very important oath—the Hippocratic oath. We swear to care for the sick in an ethical way. And we promise to do our best to prevent disease, because prevention is better than a cure. This oath comes to us from Hippocrates, who is considered one of the world's greatest physicians. Although he lived more than two millennia ago, Hippocrates had a take on medical care that I consider to be truly modern. He recognized the incredible power of food when he wrote the words, "Let food be thy medicine, and medicine be thy food."

Not that I compare myself in any way with Hippocrates, but I do wholeheartedly share his view on food: I like to think of healthy food as our very best medicine. Over and over I've seen the ability of healthy food to prevent disease, and sometimes even cure it. In my view, improving your diet can be every bit as effective as—and sometimes superior to—taking medicine. And good food doesn't cause the problematic side effects of prescription drugs.

With that in mind, no matter what amazing discoveries gut researchers make, I don't think the best "medicine" for gut health will ever come from a pill. I believe the best health comes from a diet full of foods that support the Little Buddies in your gut community. The best way to protect and support your gut microbes is to provide them with the foods that give them life.

In this section of *The Lose Your Belly Diet*, we'll focus on the many foods that nurture gut bacteria. These foods are sometimes referred to as "prebiotics" because they provide nutrients that allow gut bacteria to thrive, or as "probiotics" because they actually contain living microbes. Not only do these foods protect, support, and increase your Little Buddies, but they boost your health in numerous other ways, too. Start adding them to your daily eating plan and you'll be giving your body some of the best "medicine" available.

CHAPTER
6

Feed Your Buddies the Food
They Love Best

Your grandmother probably called it "roughage" or "bulk," but these days we refer to it as fibre. It's not trendy or sexy, but fibre is the absolute best food for gut microbes. Unfortunately, you're probably not getting nearly enough fibre in your diet, which is bad news for you and your Little Buddies.

Fibre is the word we use for a number of different types of carbohydrates found in plant foods such as fruits, vegetables, whole grains, pulses, nuts, and seeds. Your body can't really digest fibre, but your Little Buddies love it and need enough of it to thrive.

Sad to say, most Americans don't take in anywhere close to enough fibre. On average, men get about 17 grams of fibre per day, and women get about 13 grams per day—about half of what we should be having. Just to give you some perspective, you get about 17 grams of fibre by eating a cup of raspberries (8 grams), half a cup of white beans (6 grams), and one slice of whole-grain bread (3 grams).

Why don't we get the fibre we need? There are two main reasons for this. First of all, we aren't eating enough high-fibre fruits and veggies—for example, 76 percent of the US population doesn't eat enough fruit, and an astounding 87 percent of people don't eat the recommended amount of vegetables.

Fibre Guidelines for Adults

- ► Men age 50 and younger: 38 grams per day
- ► Men age 51 and older: 30 grams per day
- ► Women age 50 and younger: 25 grams per day
- ► Women age 51 and older: 21 grams per day

Second, many of the grain foods we do eat—such as white flour, sugary cereals, and white rice—are so processed that little of their natural fibre remains.

This is terrible for our Little Buddies, who live off the fibre in our diet. But it's also bad for us because a low-fibre diet is linked to a long list of health problems, as I've already mentioned, such as obesity, cardiovascular disease, type 2 diabetes, and some cancers.

I'm happy to say there's a silver lining to all this: If you haven't been getting the fibre you need, you can start to change that with your very next meal or snack. By following *The Lose Your Belly Diet*, you will add more gut-nourishing fibre to your menu every day.

Facts About Fibre

There are two primary kinds of dietary fibre: soluble and insoluble. Plant foods can have one or both kinds of fibre in them, which is why it's important to eat different kinds of high-fibre foods. Both kinds of fibre are important for good health.

Soluble fibre is found in nuts, seeds, beans, many fruits, pulses, oatmeal, and oat bran. In your body, soluble fibre dissolves in water. Eating it helps lower your blood sugar levels and your cholesterol.

Insoluble fibre doesn't dissolve in water. It is found in whole grains, seeds, and most fruits and vegetables. Its bulk helps move food through your digestive system, which helps prevent constipation, thus keeping you regular. That may not seem like a big deal, but take it from this ER doc: severe constipation sends a lot of folks to the hospital each and every day. Not only do they feel lousy, but few realize they could cure their problem simply by eating more fibre!

Both kinds of fibre pass through your gastrointestinal (GI) tract without being broken down into glucose. Instead of being digested, they remain relatively intact in your intestines, where they provide food for your Little Buddies. That's where your microbes go to work, taking out energy and nutrients for themselves but also sharing it with you.

If you don't eat enough fibre, some of your gut microbes can start to die off. Others may feed on your gut's mucus lining. This is a big problem, because when your gut's mucosal lining gets damaged, bacteria and other substances can permeate the gut. This can cause your immune system to sound the alarm and mount an inflammatory response that can harm your body, especially if it continues for a long time as chronic inflammation.

Studies in mice have found that when the fibre content in their diet is low, the layer of mucus that lines their guts gets thinner. And when mice are fed higher-fibre diets, their mucosal layer thickens. That's probably what happens in our guts, too.

We've known for a long time that eating a high-fibre diet is good for us. Studies have shown that a high-fibre diet is associated with a lower risk of heart disease, obesity, metabolic syndrome, diabetes, constipation, breast cancer, and various gastrointestinal conditions such as diverticular disease. But we haven't completely understood all of the reasons why fibre is so good for our health. Now that we're learning more about the gut microbiome, we're realizing that fibre is probably helping us stay healthy because it helps nourish and support our gut microbes.

A Dozen Easy Ways to Eat More Fibre

The average American gets less than half the recommended amount of dietary fibre. But the good news is that it's so simple to add more fibre to your diet. Here are 12 ways to start boosting your fibre intake.

1. Skip the fruit juice and eat whole fruits instead.

2. Choose whole grains instead of processed grains—for example, brown rice instead of white rice.

3. Eat whole-grain bread, pasta, cereals, and crackers instead of white bread, white pasta, and low-fibre cereal and crackers. Look for a whole grain as the first ingredient on the label.

4. In soups, chilli, and pasta sauces, replace some or all of the meat with beans or lentils.

5. Eat fruit and/or vegetables with every meal.

6. At snack time, pair raw veggies with delicious, fibre-rich dips such as guacamole, hummus, bean dip, and salsa.

7. Choose fruits and vegetables that are highest in fibre. For example, raspberries contain much more fibre (8 grams per cup) than strawberries (3 grams per cup).

8. Add beans, lentils, split peas, or seeds to your salads.

9. Experiment with new grains. You may not be familiar with amaranth, barley, bulgur, and quinoa, for example, but these grains are delicious, high in fibre, and a much better choice than white rice or white potatoes.

10. Swap mayonnaise for hummus as a sandwich spread. Hummus provides you with protein as well as fibre.

11. Instead of breadcrumbs, use ground nuts or seeds as a coating for baked fish or poultry.

12. Eat fruits and vegetables with their skin on—the skin of apples, pears, cucumbers, sweet potatoes, and other produce is an excellent source of fibre.

Here's something to keep in mind as you ramp up your fibre intake. You may notice wind, cramps, and bloating as you start adding more high-fibre foods to your diet, especially if you increase the fibre intake suddenly. Don't worry; this should be temporary—once your system gets used to the extra fibre, those symptoms should disappear. And if you increase fibre intake gradually, it's less likely to happen. Be sure to drink plenty of water, which helps fibre do its job most effectively. Smooth moves here we come!

What About Fibre Supplements?

If fibre is so good for our guts, shouldn't we be taking fibre supplements? That's a good question, but it's a question that doesn't have a final answer.

Some studies have found that taking fibre supplements can help some people lose weight. However, I believe that it's much better to get your fibre from food rather than supplements. Here's why: In addition to fibre, food

Fibre and Weight

As we discussed earlier, scientists have found links between weight and the diversity of our gut microbe communities. Overall, lean adults tend to have a greater number and diversity of bacteria species in their guts than obese people. Although we still have a lot to learn about obesity and gut bacteria, we have reason to believe that taking steps to support, nourish, and increase them could help with obesity.

This all makes sense. For years we've known that people who eat high-fibre diets tend to have more success losing weight and maintaining a healthy weight than those who eat low-fibre diets. For example, one study found that simply increasing fibre intake to 30 grams per day can lead to long-term weight loss. And many other studies have had similar results, all of which suggest that eating more fibre is a surefire way to both lose weight and keep it off.

Scientists assumed that fibre helped with weight loss because it fills you up and helps stave off hunger. But now, adding in what we're learning about fibre and gut bacteria, it's looking like there may be yet another reason that high-fibre diets help with weight loss. It's likely that in addition to filling you up and tamping down your hunger, high-fibre foods such as fruits, vegetables, whole grains, pulses, nuts, and seeds may also help bring about weight loss because they support gut bacteria that are linked to leanness. Additionally, high-fibre foods may help with weight loss by crowding highly processed, high-sugar foods that fuel obesity-linked bacteria out of the diet.

We still have a lot to learn about the connections between gut microbes and weight loss. But what it all comes down to is this: no matter what biological processes are involved, we know that high-fibre food helps you reach and maintain a healthy weight. And by following *The Lose Your Belly Diet*, you'll get all the fibre you and your Little Buddies need.

Do you hear that? I think I hear your Little Buddies having a dance party celebrating all that fibre you're going to be giving them!

provides vitamins, minerals, antioxidants, and other nutrients that are good for you and that may facilitate weight loss. And fibre supplements contain only certain types of fibre. Actual food provides all of the different types of dietary fibre we need, along with other things that scientists probably haven't even identified yet.

Highest-Fibre Foods

Food	Grams of Fibre
FRUIT	
Apple, medium, with peel	4
Blueberries, 1 cup	4
Pear, medium, with peel	6
Raspberries or blackberries, 1 cup	8
VEGETABLES	
Greens (turnip, mustard, spring, Swiss chard, beetroot), 1 cup cooked	4–5
Peas, 1 cup cooked	9
Broccoli, 1 cup	5
Artichoke, 1 medium cooked	10
Summer squash, 1 cup cooked	5
Acorn squash, 1 cup cooked	9
GRAINS	
Whole-grain bread, 1 slice	2–3
Bran or other very high-fibre cereal, ¾ cup	6–10
Air-popped popcorn, 3 cups	4
Cooked barley, ½ cup	3
Cooked bulgur, ½ cup	4
PULSES	
Beans (black, kidney, pinto, cannellini, white), ½ cup cooked	6–9.5
Butterbeans, ½ cup cooked	7
Chickpeas, ½ cup cooked	6
Lentils, ½ cup cooked	8
Split peas, ½ cup cooked	8
NUTS AND SEEDS	
Nuts (almonds, pistachios, cashews, peanuts, walnuts) 30g, or nut butter, 2 tablespoons	2–4
Flaxseed, 30g	8

There's no harm in considering fibre supplements such as psyllium and methylcellulose. Keep this in mind, though: they can interfere with the absorption of certain medications, so if you take any medication you should check with your doctor or pharmacist before using fibre supplements. For people who don't bother eating a high-fibre diet, fibre supplements can be a good choice. But I think it is way better for you and your microbes to get your fibre from food.

Coming Up

In the next few chapters, we'll look at the many foods that provide a bundle of gut-nurturing fibre. They're all included in *The Lose Your Belly Diet*, because they all feed your gut in important ways. We'll start with a group of foods that are so good for your Little Buddies that I refer to them as "Prebiotic Superstars."

CHAPTER
7

Fill Your Belly with Prebiotic Superstars

Prebiotic foods are those that best support your Little Buddies. These foods are referred to as prebiotics (pre = "before" and biotic = "life") because they are fantastic sources of the soluble and insoluble fibre that literally give life to your microbes by providing the nourishment they need to survive. Fruits and vegetables are among the best prebiotic foods, which is why I think of them as Prebiotic Superstars that are included in nearly all of the meals and snacks in *The Lose Your Belly Diet*.

Why are they so beneficial? It starts once again with fibre. Fruits and veggies are packed with fibre—for example, a cup of sweet little raspberries provides 8 grams of fibre, and a cup of chopped carrots has 4 grams. But when it comes to fibre and your personal microbiome, the numbers tell only part of the story.

Sure, you're aiming to eat a high number of grams of fibre every day. But there are various kinds of fibre, and your gut bacteria need them all. In fact, like you and me, different kinds of bacteria each have their favourite kinds of dietary fibre. Eating a wide range of plant foods—especially fruits and vegetables—is the best way to give all of them the nutrients that allow them to flourish. No single fruit or vegetable provides you with all of the nutrients you need, so it's important to eat a mix of fruits and vegetables (as well as pulses, nuts, and whole grains) to make sure you get all of the types of fibre your Little Buddies love.

For example, a type of fibre known as inulin, which is found in onions, beetroot, and chicory, is a big favourite for some types of gut microbes. Another is pectin, which is found in various fruits such as apples and berries. And mushrooms provide a fibre known as mannan, which some of your Little Buddies love to live on. So, by eating a large selection of fruits and vegetables—as well as other high-fibre grains, pulses, and seeds—you give your Little Buddies a fantastic buffet of life-supporting nutrients.

A Cornucopia of Benefits

People who eat plenty of produce tend to have a more diverse gut microbe community. Overall, when researchers check out the gut microbes in volunteers who eat larger amounts of fruits and vegetables, they tend to have more diversity than those who eat lesser amounts of fruits and vegetables.

In addition to being high in fibre, fruits and vegetables serve up an enormous range of disease-fighting nutrients, including potassium, folate (also known as folic acid), vitamin A, and vitamin C. These and other nutrients help reduce the risk of heart attacks, stroke, cardiovascular disease, type 2 diabetes, obesity, certain eye diseases, and some kinds of cancer.

There's actually a pretty dramatic connection between produce and health. For example, researchers compiling the results of many large studies have found that people who eat more than five servings per day of fruits and vegetables have about a 20 percent lower risk of coronary heart disease and stroke than people who eat fewer than three servings per day. Think about it: a 20 percent lower risk. There aren't many drugs that can boast success rates like that—but it's business as usual for the berries, apples, broccoli, cabbage, spinach, and other delicious fruits and vegetables that we can easily include in our diets every day without any of the side effects of powerful cardiovascular medications.

The conventional wisdom for fruits and vegetables is to "eat from the rainbow" by including many different colours of produce in your diet. Some of the antioxidants in produce are actually the compounds that give fruits and vegetables their bright colours—for example, lutein, the deep-yellow pigment that gives corn, carrots, and other vegetables their yellowish-orange hue, is an antioxidant that boosts eye health by helping to reduce the risk of age-related macular degeneration and cataracts. (Lutein is also found in various green veggies

Going Organic

Unfortunately, conventionally grown fruits and vegetables are raised with large amounts of pesticides. Although there hasn't been an enormous amount of research on this yet, I suspect there are connections between damage to gut microbes and the use of pesticides and synthetic fertilizers. For this reason, I think it's best to choose organic produce whenever possible. For tips on buying organic food (and fitting it into your budget), see chapter 11.

as well.) By eating produce that's red, dark green, yellow, orange, blue, and purple, you are sure to get a good range of health-boosting antioxidants—the ones we know about, as well as the ones that haven't yet been discovered.

It's also a good idea to eat the vegetables that some researchers think of as being extra useful to gut bacteria because of the types of fibre they contain: asparagus, carrots, garlic, Jerusalem artichokes, turnips, leeks, onions, radishes, and tomatoes.

Generally, raw produce is better for your gut microbes than cooked, because cooking breaks down some of the complex carbohydrates in foods. When fruits and veggies are eaten raw (or lightly cooked), they are more likely to be broken down lower in the GI tract—down in the large intestine, where most of your Little Buddies live. I'm not saying you should never eat cooked veggies—even when they're cooked, vegetables deliver great value to your body as well as your Buddies. But the more raw veggies you can tuck into your daily diet, the better off your Little Buddies will be. Leave the skin on vegetables such as courgettes, aubergines, and tomatoes rather than peeling it off. And don't forget about the seeds in tomatoes, cucumbers, and other seed-bearing veggies. Seeds and skin typically contain lots of fibre.

Raw Veggie Tips

Fruits and vegetables are both an important part of a gut-healthy diet. It's usually not hard to convince people to eat fruit—just about everyone loves these sweet treats. Vegetables can be a tougher sell even though there is no downside to eating lots and lots of vegetables.

Dr. T's Tasty Tip

If you are someone who is always bored with your salad, I understand! I've been there; I used to hate salads. Try using hummus or guacamole on your salad instead of salad dressing. Both are delicious and packed with nutrients.

I admit it: I am not a natural-born veggie eater. I grew up in the Midwest, where meat and gravy occupied most of the plate, and overcooked vegetables sat well to the side, usually in a pool of butter. Even now I am not someone who gravitates naturally to raw veggies in their naked, unadorned form. I'm happy to gobble up fruit, but veggies—especially raw veggies—aren't something I typically crave. But because I know how important they are for me, I've figured out a few fun tips that have helped me get the raw veggies I need.

Great-tasting dips are one of my veggie tips. No matter how nutritionally virtuous it is, a bowl of raw veggies bores me. But if I have a delicious dip to scoot my veggies in before I munch them, I can mow them up happily. There's nothing like hummus, guacamole, salsa, tahini, or yogurt dip to convert raw veggies from an obligation into an enjoyable snack. To help you get your veggies down, I've included recipes for lots of quick, tasty dips in the recipe section of this book—be sure to try my Cool Cucumber Yogurt Dip, Creamy Avocado White Bean Dip, and Mediterranean Ricotta Dip. And every one of my salad dressings—from Simple Vinaigrette to Lime Mint Dressing to Tahini—can moonlight as a fantastic dip for raw veggies.

Throughout this book I'll be sharing some of my other favourite tips as well. They are quick ways to add flavour and fun to your meals!

Chow, Baby

Here's another veggie tip: a fun, simple-to-make dish called chow-chow.

Chow-chow is a type of relish that you're probably familiar with if you grew up in the American South or parts of the Midwest or even Canada. Families made it at home with the bounty from their vegetable gardens. Usually it would be preserved in Mason jars and stored in the pantry or basement and eaten throughout the autumn and winter months. The vegetables used for chow-chow included just about anything that grew in the family vegetable garden or on the local farm—red or green tomatoes, cabbage, onions, carrots, cauliflower, broccoli, corn, peppers, asparagus, green beans, peas, you name it.

Chow-chow was commonly served as a condiment or side dish with meat, poultry, fish, or other foods. Traditionally, chow-chow was pickled, meaning the vegetables were soaked in salty water (brine) and then cooked with vinegar, herbs, spices, and sweeteners.

Traditional chow-chow usually contains a huge amount of sugar, and the veggies in it are cooked. I wanted a chow-chow that would be friendlier to my Little Buddies, filled with lots of the raw veggies that support gut microbes so well, but without the sugar. The result is *Lose Your Belly* Chow-Chow, which represents an evolution of the traditional veggie relish.

Lose Your Belly Chow-Chow replaces cooked veggies with raw veggies, because our gut bacteria love all the fibre in raw veggies. And instead of sugar, my chow-chow recipes feature fresh herbs, savoury spices, tangy citrus, and other bright tastes that combine with the natural flavour of the vegetables to create a fresh, delicious side dish or snack that will make you and your gut happy.

Lose Your Belly Chow-Chow is an incredibly versatile, fibre-rich food. It's a great go-to side for main-dish proteins. You can also toss it over greens to make an instant salad, spoon it into burritos or tacos, use it as a topping for open sandwiches or veggie burgers, or eat it straight out of the bowl. It even tastes good spooned over omelettes. Chow-chow travels well and makes an easy addition to a packed lunch or picnic. To turn it into a snack, pair it with hummus and whole-grain crackers; or make it a meal by adding in beans, nuts, olives, chopped avocado, shredded chicken, flaked tuna, or whatever else you have on hand.

I include several chow-chow recipes in the recipe section of this book. Follow them as written, or use them as a starting point to create your own chow-chows using the vegetables and fresh herbs that catch your eye at the supermarket or greengrocer. Vary the flavour by choosing different kinds of oil (walnut, sesame, avocado, etc.), vinegar, herbs, and spices. Heck, you can even throw in some fruit if you want—a handful of berries, maybe, or chopped apple or pear. It's all good.

Plants in a Cup

Here's good news for coffee lovers: microbiome research suggests that drinking coffee is good for your gut microbes. Moderation is best, since coffee contains caffeine that can cause jitters and insomnia in some people. Stick to no more than about 950ml of coffee daily—the amount that delivers about 400 milligrams of caffeine—or less if it bothers you. Tea is fine also, as is wine in moderation—probably because these beverages are plant-based, and we know how much our Little Buddies love real food!

And to make any chow-chow recipe even more interesting (and good for your Little Buddies), feel free to mix in ½ cup of kimchi or live-culture sauerkraut per serving. I'll explain more later.

One of the great things about chow-chow is that it offers you an opportunity to use some of the new vegetables you buy at the farmer's market but aren't quite sure what to do with when you get home. And it's a nice way to use up vegetables from your own garden that grow in large quantities—I'm talking about you, courgettes. It also gives you cover if you want to sneak in vegetables that people don't like. A friend of mine whose son claims to detest summer squash eats it readily when it's hidden among the veggies he likes in Summer Harvest Chow-Chow.

Make sure to chop, dice, or shred the veggies into small pieces so the chow-chow is easily spooned. If you need a little sweetness, add just a drop of honey, although I think you'll find that with all the other bold flavours, you won't need sweetener. Chow-chow stays fresh in the refrigerator for a few days, so make a big batch and you'll be all set.

A Big Bar of Salad Tips

I am a huge salad bar fan. I travel a lot, and instead of heading to restaurants I often make my way to a supermarket instead. Many have salad bars, and some have exceptional salad bars. So, instead of eating a gut bomb meal at a restaurant, I have an awesome salad from the supermarket. Not only do I get better food, but I usually save money, too!

This isn't some plain old lettuce and dressing salad—it's a superstar salad! Here are some of my tips for getting the best from a supermarket salad bar.

Go for the greens. Start your salad with a layer of greens—spinach, Swiss chard, kale, lettuces, mustard greens, whatever's available. Avoid the bland iceberg lettuce—go for deep colour in your greens!

Pour on dressing—judiciously. If you want your greens lightly coated with salad dressing, add it now and toss the greens around a bit to disperse it. Choose a dressing made with extra-virgin olive oil, avocado oil, or other healthy fat. You can't measure it in the shop, but keep an eye on the serving size to avoid going overboard—aim for no more than two tablespoons of dressing total. I personally use about a tablespoon of olive oil and a tablespoon of vinegar. I dress my greens first and then pile on other ingredients. Needless to say, skip the fat-laden creamy dressings altogether.

Top the greens with more veggies. Cherry tomatoes, sliced peppers, mushrooms, broccoli, cauliflower—pile them on. Look for roasted veggies, too—some bars offer roasted aubergine, summer squash, or other veggies.

Add in whole grains. Look for quinoa, bulgur, tabbouleh, brown rice, or wild rice. They add fibre, protein, and a delicious nutty flavour.

Pick your protein. Most salad bars have black beans, kidney beans, or—if you're lucky—a spicy three-bean salad studded with onions and garlic. These add protein and fibre to your salad. Other good protein sources are hard-boiled eggs, sliced baked chicken, or plain tuna.

Toss in nuts and seeds. Almonds, peanuts, cashews, and other nuts add protein and fibre, as do seeds such as sesame, pumpkin, and sunflower.

Don't forget fruit! If you're lucky enough to find chopped fresh fruit at your salad bar, sprinkle it on for an extra burst of sweetness. Avoid or go light on dried fruit, though, because it's usually high in sugar and calories.

Sprinkle on a little cheese. If you like, toss in a small amount of cheese, such as crumbled feta or blue cheese.

Dr. T's Tasty Tip

The secret to a successful salad, in my humble opinion, is in the "toss." Making sure a salad is tossed well, with all the ingredients combined, ensures a flavourful, enjoyable salad. Make sure to use a bowl that's big enough for tossing!

Or, sprinkle on nutritional yeast. It's yeast, but it has an enjoyable cheesy flavour—plus, it contains vitamin B12 and protein.

Stud your salad with healthy fats. I usually add in olives, avocado, or guacamole, but obviously be aware that calories can add up fast even from healthy fats.

Avoid the gut bombs. Skip over the junky foods that shouldn't even be on the salad bar that will turn your healthy salad into a heavy meal. Avoid gut bombs such as deep-fried noodles (or anything deep-fried), croutons, tortilla crisps, imitation bacon bits (why do they even exist?), and mayonnaise-laden potato salad, pasta salad, tuna salad, and egg salad.

Now, step back. If you're like me, you may sometimes build a salad that's bigger than you need. Eat the right amount and save the rest for a snack—or better yet, tomorrow's lunch!

Coming Up

Next up in the parade of super-healthy foods is a family of foods that you probably know well—although maybe you haven't been paying enough attention to some of its less well-known members. Don't worry: I'll reintroduce you in the next chapter.

CHAPTER

8

Pick Plenty of Plant Protein

Ask people to name a protein food and they're most likely to say meat. Ask again and they'll probably add some other animal foods to the list: chicken, fish, shellfish, eggs, and dairy. Maybe on the third try they'll get around to mentioning the protein foods that actually are the best for your Little Buddies: pulses, soya, nuts, and seeds. These high-protein foods tend to be left off the list because they come from plants rather than animals.

I sometimes think of plant proteins as the forgotten proteins. When news breaks about studies showing positive connections between protein and weight loss, for example, the images accompanying those reports are typically of juicy steaks, roasted chicken, or even fatty bacon. Rarely are the images of plant proteins. That's a shame, because plant proteins are so good for you and your gut microbes that they should be appearing on your plate on a regular basis.

Don't worry: I'm not going to recommend that you become a vegan or even a vegetarian—unless you want to, that is. And I think eggs and dairy are very good protein sources. What I am suggesting, though, is that you replace some of the meat in your diet with plant proteins. That's the best way to get the protein you need while giving your Little Buddies even more of the fibre they love.

Protein and Health

First, a quick review of protein's role in nutrition. Protein helps maintain the health of our skin, muscles, organs, blood, and just about every other body part. Without adequate protein, we can't live, and we definitely can't thrive. Protein is made up of chains of amino acids. Although our bodies can manufacture some amino acids, others—which are known as "essential" amino acids—must come from food.

As a baseline, we need between 46 and 56 grams of protein per day. But if you're trying to lean up, adding some extra protein to your diet makes sense, because protein helps chase away hunger and leaves you feeling fuller longer. Studies have found that including protein in meals makes them more satisfying because it helps curb post-meal hunger, especially when it's combined with high-fibre vegetables, fruits, and whole grains. Protein appears to have an effect on hormones such as ghrelin, which is referred to as the "hunger hormone," and leptin, known as the "satiety hormone." By including protein in meals and snacks, you help set the stage for your hormones to do their jobs most effectively, so you don't feel overly hungry and so you do feel satiated after eating. For those reasons, I recommend that you pack protein into most, if not all, of your meals and snacks—as I do in my own life and in *The Lose Your Belly Diet*.

Protein also plays a part in keeping blood sugar stable. When you eat a meal or snack with a moderate amount of protein and fibre, your blood sugar levels go up and come down gradually, which is exactly what you want because it's the best thing for your body and your hunger. But when you eat a snack or meal that is low in protein and high in fast-burning sugar and low-quality carbohydrates, your blood sugar zooms up, then falls rapidly, leaving you ravenous for more food long before your next meal or snack. That's not where you want to be.

Dr. T's Time-Saving Tip

To save time cooking eggs, spray a microwave-safe bowl with cooking spray, crack eggs into the bowl, and microwave until fully cooked.

You can get protein from plant foods and animal foods. Both are good, but plant proteins are especially beneficial for two reasons: because of what they *do* contain, and because of what they *don't* contain.

A Jackpot of Nutrients

Let's start with what plant-based protein foods *do* contain. When you eat plant proteins such as beans, nuts, or seeds, you're not just getting protein—you're also getting a big dose of something I rave about all book long as the food our Little Buddies love most: dietary fibre.

For example, ½ cup of cooked black beans has 7 grams of protein *plus* 7.5 grams of fibre; ½ cup of cooked lentils has 9 grams of protein *plus* 8 grams of fibre; 30 grams of almonds has 6 grams of protein *plus* 4 grams of fibre. You get the idea—when you eat meat, you just get the protein. But when you eat plant-based proteins, you get protein *plus* fibre.

And there's more: In addition to vitamins and minerals, plant-based proteins also contain a huge range of antioxidants, such as flavonoids, carotenoids, polyphenols, phenolic acids, and other compounds that can help prevent cellular damage, lower cancer risk, and help reduce inflammation in the body.

Eating plant proteins can go a long way toward reducing your risk of various kinds of diseases. Take nuts, for example. There's been a lot of research about nuts and health, but I can sum up their findings with a single quote from Dr. Frank Hu, a professor of nutrition and epidemiology at the Harvard T. H. Chan School of Public Health. Dr. Hu is one of the researchers who has worked on the long-running Nurses' Health Study and Physicians' Health Study, which have tracked the eating habits of more than 130,000 people for over three decades. After publishing one of the many articles reporting findings from the two study groups, Dr. Hu said this: "We found that people who ate nuts every day lived longer, healthier lives than people who didn't eat nuts." Dr. Hu went on to say that people in the studies who ate nuts were less likely to die of cancer, heart disease, and respiratory disease—in fact, they were 20 percent less likely to die of *anything* during the course of the study than people who didn't eat nuts. And that isn't even mentioning nuts' association with a lower body weight.

Talk about letting food be your medicine—good luck finding a prescription medication that is as effective as nuts! And if you do find one, I can guarantee

---

Dr. T's Takeout Tip

If it's one of those days and takeout is the only option—or if you're travelling and need a quick meal—aim for a place where you can pick and choose what you want in your meal. If you choose a burrito bowl or salad with brown rice, black and pinto beans, veggies, salsa, and guacamole, it can actually be a decent meal, just don't overdo it. Leftovers are always great! Thai food and other ethnic foods are fun options, provided you stay away from noodle dishes and instead opt for the veggie-heavy dishes.

---

you, it will have big-time side effects (and won't be nearly as enjoyable or inexpensive as a handful of almonds, walnuts, or cashews).

Pulses are another great source of plant-based protein. Pulses include beans, peas, lentils, and soybeans. (Technically, peanuts are also pulses, but most people consider them nuts, so that's how I think of them.) Pulses are an amazing source of fibre as well as protein. As with nuts, there are many studies that delineate the benefits of beans and other pulses. Eating them on a regular basis is associated with a lower risk of heart disease, diabetes, some kinds of cancer, and obesity. When researchers look at pulses' connection to weight loss, the findings make them smile. And I smile, too, when I hear about studies like the one that found that obese men who included pulses in their diets lost 50 percent more weight than those who didn't. If that doesn't turn you on to beans, I don't know what will. There's a reason I eat nuts and beans virtually every single day.

Questionable Compounds

Now, let's look at what you *don't* get when you eat plant protein: namely, the compounds in meats that may raise disease risk. (Red meat includes any meat from mammals, including beef, lamb, goat, veal, venison, and pork, which despite what its advertisers say, is not "the other white meat.") For example, red meat contains carnitine, a compound that has been linked to atherosclerosis, or clogged arteries. And conventionally raised red meat may have hormones, antibiotics, and other ingredients that aren't good for us or our Little Buddies. When researchers look closely at the long-term health

---

Dr. T's Time-Saving Tip

For a quick lunch, have a veggie burger topped with sauerkraut and regular or whole-grain mustard. Or mix canned tuna with hummus, olive oil, and black pepper and spread on a slice of whole-grain bread. Yum!

---

outlook of people who eat a lot of red meat, the news isn't great. For example, Harvard researchers have found that eating too much red meat may be associated with higher rates of heart disease, stroke, type 2 diabetes, some forms of cancer, excess weight/obesity, and early death from various causes.

I grew up eating meat at just about every meal, but I have to tell you, the more I have learned to embrace the ease of preparing foods like black beans, the less meat I eat. These days, I consider myself a flexitarian, which means that although I do eat some red meat, I get most of my protein from plant foods, eggs, and dairy. I'll eat an occasional steak, but to tell you the truth, I'm really just as happy with a tasty veggie burger (I'll give examples later), a healthy bean burrito, or a bowl of chilli.

In fact, I rarely bring meat into my house—my go-to meals at home are all centred on plant-based proteins, which I find to be so much easier to store and prepare than meat. I do eat meat sometimes in restaurants, but on a daily basis I'd say I'm 90-plus percent vegetarian. Meat does provide certain nutrients, and sometimes I find myself craving a burger and won't shy away from it. That's why I recommend a mix-and-match approach as the healthiest way to get the widest variety of proteins and nutrients, and it's why I've designed *The Lose Your Belly Diet* in a way that makes it easy for you to include all kinds of plant proteins in your daily meal plan.

Not a Cure

Processed meat is the one I really worry about. (Processed meat includes bacon, ham, sausage, pepperoni, hot dogs, jerky, canned meat, cured meat, smoked meat, and even the lunch meats at your supermarket's deli counter, such as salami, roast beef, and turkey.) Based on its analysis of the current research on processed meat, the World Health Organization (WHO) considers it to be carcinogenic (that is, cancer-causing) to humans. WHO and other health organizations lean heavily in favour of minimizing the processed meat in your diet—and I have to say, I agree with them 100 percent.

Again, I'll point to Harvard studies of more than 130,000 adults to give you an idea of the impact of red meat and processed meat on health. After tracking volunteers' diets for up to 32 years, researchers found that people who eat greater amounts of red meat and processed meat are more likely to die early from heart disease, cancer, and other diseases than those who eat less red meat and processed meat. For example, regularly eating red meat was linked with a 50 percent increase in type 2 diabetes risk.

We don't know for sure that meat is the only factor in raising disease risk in these studies. Frequent meat eaters may have other health habits that influence their risk, although researchers do try to control for things like smoking, sedentary behaviour, and other factors. But even then, there is definitely a smoking gun when it comes to meat eating—or perhaps I should call it a smoking barbecue.

Here's something else to keep in mind: studies that find connections between disease and meat consumption are typically done with conventionally raised meat from animals dosed with synthetic hormones, antibiotics, and diets that are designed to fatten them up fast. I believe that organic meat from grass-fed animals is healthier than conventional meat, even if I don't have a pile of studies to point to as proof. It just makes sense to me that meat raised in a more healthful way would be better for us than conventionally raised meat. I actually believe eating meat in moderation from animals raised in a more natural way may turn out to be healthy for us. For that reason, when I eat a steak or a burger, I go with organic, grass-fed meat. It costs more but in the long run you actually save money because you are eating it less.

And remember this: grilling can add cancer-causing compounds to meat, so opt for baking, sautéing, poaching, stir-frying, and braising as much as possible. Honestly, whenever I read a study about meat, I'm reminded of the fact that it can be such a high-maintenance choice in terms of potential harm to our health and to the planet, not to mention the amount of time it takes to prepare it! That's precisely why at home I'll choose a bean/quinoa veggie burger with a pile of fixings over a meat burger almost every time.

Coming Up

Now, it's time to start eating some favourite foods that health "experts" have spent years telling us to avoid. Don't listen to them, folks—it's time to start eating grains again. More about that in the next chapter.

CHAPTER
9

Don't Give Up on Grains!

No food group has been more maligned during the past few years than grains. So-called diet "experts" have turned people against grains, urging them to follow fad diets that contain few or no grains. I never understood this, because I always believed whole grains could be an important staple in a healthy diet. I figured that like all fads, this one would burn itself out, and that is exactly what seems to be happening lately. The tide is turning back, and people are beginning to rediscover the nutritional benefits of grains.

I attribute a lot of my good health (GI and otherwise) to whole grains, so I'm thrilled to be able to help bring grains back to the table! For me one of the biggest benefits of grains is how filling they are—when my meal includes a dose of healthy whole grains, I can count on my hunger and taste buds being well satiated!

Now, when I talk about "grains," I'm referring to whole grains, not refined grains.

Whole grains are good for us, but refined grains are pretty much the opposite. Whole grains are made up of the entire seed, or kernel, of a plant. The seed consists of the germ, the bran, and the endosperm, and whole-grain foods contain all of those components. With refined grains, the healthy parts of the plant's seed are stripped away. Foods such as white bread, white pasta, white rice, white flour, and other refined grains have had most of their nutrient-rich bran and germ removed. Thus, almost all of its protein, fibre, vitamins, and minerals are lost. The main things left in a refined grain are simple carbohydrates that act much like sugar in the body. But when a grain is left whole, it provides a nice mix of important nutrients, especially ones that benefit your gut microbes.

As we've discussed, your Little Buddies love fibre, and whole grains are a great place to get it. So in this chapter, we'll take a look at how grains contribute to gut health and ways to incorporate whole grains into your daily eating plan.

Grains and Health

As human microbiome researchers look more closely at what helps and harms our gut microbes, they are discovering that whole grains have a really important role to play in gut health. For example, in one study, researchers asked volunteers to eat whole-grain barley and brown rice each day for four weeks. When they analyzed the volunteers' faecal samples, they found a noticeable increase in the diversity of their microbes. And, not surprisingly—to me, anyway—the volunteers had lower levels of inflammation and blood glucose.

In another study, volunteers were placed on two different diets for three weeks: one that was high in whole grains and one that was low in whole grains. After eating the diet that was high in whole grains, volunteers had a significant increase in the diversity of their gut microbes compared to the diet that was low in whole grains. And, although both diets had the same number of calories, the people following the diet that was high in whole grains lost more weight and body fat than those who ate few whole grains—and they weren't even *trying* to lose weight. That's what I call a success!

Other studies have found an impressive connection between whole grains and heart health. For example, Harvard researchers analyzing the eating habits of some 75,000 women in the Nurses' Health Study found that those who ate two to three servings a day of whole grains were 30 percent less likely to die from heart disease or have a heart attack during a 10-year follow-up period than women who rarely ate whole grains. Let me tell you: I'm an emergency room doctor, and I see a lot of people with heart disease and heart attacks. The idea of being able to reduce the risk of such a savage disease simply by eating whole grains is pretty phenomenal.

Various studies have found that whole grains even seem to help protect against diabetes. For example, an 18-year study of 160,000 women found that

Whole Grains on the Menu	

Here are some of the delicious whole grains you can add to your daily diet:

Amaranth	Millet
Barley	Oats
Brown rice	Quinoa
Buckwheat	Rye
Bulgur	Spelt
Corn (including whole-grain cornmeal and popcorn)	Teff
	Triticale
Cracked wheat	Wheat
Farro	Wild rice

those who ate two to three servings a day of whole grains were 30 percent less likely to develop type 2 diabetes than those who ate few to no whole grains. Thirty percent is a pretty amazing drop in risk, especially for something as easy as a change in diet.

And one of my favourite studies is the one that looked at the results of 45 other studies (researchers refer to this as a "meta-analysis") and found that whole-grain intake is associated with a lower risk of a very long list of diseases and health conditions, from heart disease and cancer to infectious diseases and respiratory diseases.

Ladies and gentlemen of the jury, we have a verdict: it's time to put whole grains back on our plates.

I could spend the next 10 pages telling you about studies that have found good stuff about whole grains. But I don't think you feel like reading all that—and as for me, I'd rather tell you about how delicious whole-grain foods are. I honestly don't think I could stomach a healthy diet for a lifetime without them.

Give Grains a Try

In general, we don't have a lot of experience with whole grains. Maybe you eat whole-wheat bread sometimes, and perhaps you have oatmeal for breakfast or popcorn at the movies. But there's a big world of whole

What Is Sprouted Grain Bread?

You may have noticed loaves of sprouted grain bread in the shops. These are breads made with whole grains that have started to sprout. Once the sprout grows, the grains and sprouts are ground into flour. The advantage of sprouting is that it is said to allow the release of enzymes that make it easier for the grain's nutrients to be absorbed by the body. These breads are loaded with fibre, protein, and flavour.

grains out there that many people have never even tried. If you're one of those people, I want to invite you to give these yummy grains a try.

My recommendation is to start experimenting with quinoa, because I consider it one of the most accessible of all whole grains, and because it's so easy to cook. Quinoa—pronounced KEEN-wah—is a plant grown in South America, particularly in the Peruvian Andes, that is sometimes referred to as "the mother grain." (Although the part of the quinoa plant that we eat is a seed, the plant itself is a grain, so we refer to quinoa as a grain.) Quinoa is a rich source of nutrients—for example, it contains all nine of the essential amino acids, which makes it a complete plant protein. It also contains several B vitamins, as well as iron, magnesium, manganese, phosphorus, and other minerals. And it has antioxidants, which are compounds that lower inflammation and may reduce the risk of inflammatory diseases.

But most importantly for your Little Buddies, quinoa contains fibre—about 3 grams in a half-cup serving. And it's a popular grain among people who avoid gluten, either because of coeliac disease or gluten intolerance.

A lot of people like the way quinoa tastes plain—it has a chewy, nutty, toasty flavour by itself. (It comes in white, red, and black versions, each of which has a slightly different flavour.) What I love most about quinoa is that when you incorporate it into a dish, it does an amazingly great job of flattering the flavours of whatever else is in the dish. For example, in the Quinoa-Stuffed Peppers recipe I include in this book, the quinoa takes on the Southwestern flavours of the peppers, tomatoes, cumin, and chilli powder. But in the Quinoa Veggie Pilaf, the nuttiness of the quinoa enhances the earthy flavours of the vegetables. Quinoa is like the perfect party guest: it gets along with everyone, but doesn't have to be the centre of attention.

Quinoa is also a great ingredient in just about any salad because it supports rather than takes over the flavours of the vegetables, salad dressing, and other ingredients. It makes a fine substitute for rice or pasta in Asian, Indian, or Italian dishes. And it is a nice addition to a chilli or soup that needs a little extra substance to it.

This versatile grain is as easy to cook as rice. You combine it with water, bring the water to a boil, cover the pot, and simmer it until the water is absorbed—usually about 15 minutes. (You can also make it in a rice cooker and there are frozen versions that only require a microwave.) Then, all you do is fluff it and it's ready to eat. Serve quinoa plain as a side dish or mixed with vegetables, herbs, or spices. Or, to make it the centre of a quinoa salad, let it cool and then toss it with salad dressing, chopped fresh vegetables, nuts, seeds, and even chopped fresh fruit. It really is one of the most adaptable ingredients in the kitchen.

Once you get comfortable with quinoa, try cooking with other grains, too. Some of them take a bit longer to prepare or have stronger flavours, but once you know how to cook them you will appreciate their flexibility and their delicious taste. Believe me, when you start eating whole grains, you'll be amazed at how bland white rice tastes!

Barley is another great grain to try. High in fibre and nutrients, barley is, like quinoa, an excellent stand-in for white rice and is a welcome addition to soups, stews, and salads. Barley takes longer to cook than quinoa, but it's worth the wait.

You can also get whole grains from breads, cereals, granolas, oatmeal, crackers, tortillas, and pasta. Be sure to check the label and make sure that a whole grain is the first ingredient. In the case of cereals, granolas, oatmeal, and breads, check for sweeteners as well—if sugar, high-fructose corn syrup, or other sweeteners are early on the list of ingredients, you may want to choose a different product with less sugar.

Breakfast Grains

Picking high-fibre cereal, granola, or oatmeal can be tricky. As mentioned, many contain a lot of sugar or other sweeteners, and granola tends to have

Dr. T's Time-Saving Tip

Although whole grains can take a while to cook, they're actually one of the best fast foods ever. That's because you can cook them in quantity and freeze them for future use. (Or you can buy them precooked and microwave ready.) Here's my favourite whole-grain tip: I always have precooked quinoa, barley, and brown rice in my freezer. Just a couple of minutes in the microwave, and they're ready to serve as a side dish or to mix into salads, chilli, burritos, enchiladas, pilafs, or soups.

Try this: Cook up a big pot of grains. When they're fully cooled, scoop half-cup portions into a cupcake baking pan sprayed with nonstick baking spray. Stick the pan in the freezer, and when the grains are frozen, pop them out of the pan and into a big plastic bag, which you can store back in the freezer. Then, when you need a serving of grains, grab one from the bag, toss it in the microwave, and heat it up for a minute or two. Voila—you'll have a serving of delicious whole grains in less time than it takes to make instant rice.

a lot of calories. So be sure to read labels, and make sure you know what you're getting.

Oats are an excellent grain to include in your diet. Not only are they good for your Little Buddies, but they also help lower the risk of heart disease by improving cholesterol levels due to a soluble fibre called beta glucan. Unfortunately, choosing oats in the supermarket can be tricky. Different kinds of oats are processed in different ways. Overall, it's best to go with oats that are the least processed. Although all whole-grain oatmeal starts out with oat grain kernels, the more processing they receive, the less interesting they are to your Little Buddies. Gut microbes like to be able to sink their teeth into oats and other grains. Here's a quick guide to the kinds of oats you'll see in shops.

Groats: The full, uncut oat grain kernel.

Steel-cut oats: Oat grain kernels cut into larger pieces with metal blades. They're also called Irish oatmeal.

Dr. T's Healthy Tip

Instead of granola, which can be high in calories and sugar, choose a high-fibre cereal. It'll get your Little Buddies dancing early in the a.m.

Scottish oats: Oat grain kernels that are stone-ground into smaller pieces.

Rolled oats: Also referred to as old-fashioned oats, these are made when oat grain kernels are steamed and then rolled into flakes. Rolled oats come in regular, quick, or instant varieties, based on how much steaming and rolling they've undergone—regular oats get the least steaming and rolling, and instant oats the most.

I recommend steel-cut oats or Scottish oats for your morning oatmeal. They are less processed than rolled oats, so they leave more for your gut microbes to feast on. Groats are even less processed than steel-cut or Scottish oats, but they take a long time to cook and aren't to everyone's taste. If you choose rolled oats, go with regular rolled rather than quick or instant. And skip the highly sweetened instant oatmeal. You and your belly don't need all that extra sugar.

It's easy to cook oatmeal from scratch with either water or milk. Cook it on the hob or in the slow cooker. And to save time, freeze cooked oatmeal in single servings, and heat it up in the microwave for a fast breakfast.

Add flavour to plain oatmeal with a sprinkle of cinnamon, nutmeg, or allspice. If you can't eat it without sweetener, drizzle in a touch of honey or molasses. Oatmeal is also delicious with chopped fruit and nuts tossed in.

Coming Up

There's one more kind of food that's great for your gut—not because of the nutrients in it, but because it actually delivers living bacteria to your gut. In the next chapter, I'll tell you all about eating, preparing, and buying probiotic foods.

CHAPTER
10

Get Your Buddies to Go

In the previous few chapters, we talked about the foods that support and nourish gut bacteria. But there are also foods that actually *contain* living microbes. Sounds kind of weird, but it's true: some foods have what's referred to as "live and active cultures" that deliver living microbes directly into your body. These foods are referred to as "probiotic foods" or "living foods."

When you eat probiotic foods, which are teeming with helpful microbes, you introduce new guests to the microbe party in your gut. As part of *The Lose Your Belly Diet*, I recommend that you include at least one probiotic food in your daily menu each day.

The live bacteria in probiotic foods help replenish microbes in the gut. Makes sense, right? If you're low on beneficial gut bacteria, you can send in some reinforcements via the probiotic foods you eat. To make sure these living things survive the digestion process, researchers have analyzed the faeces of people who eat probiotic foods such as yogurt. (Another unpleasant task, but an important one!) These studies have found that the Little Buddies in food can indeed stay alive during their journey through the digestive system.

Yogurt is the most well-known probiotic food, but there are many others as well. You may not be familiar with them, but as we learn more about the importance of having a diverse, thriving gut microbe community, they are becoming more popular. Not too long ago, you could find foods like kefir, kimchi, or kombucha only in the dark corners of health food shops or ethnic markets. But now they're increasingly available—much to my surprise, I recently came across kombucha in a supermarket. Meanwhile, probiotic foods are appearing in mainstream shops as well.

Chilling helps keep probiotic bacteria alive, so when you're looking for these foods in shops, check the refrigerated sections. They used to be tucked away in a corner, although lately I'm noticing them much more front and centre than in the past. In fact, my local shop in Nashville has a refrigerated case dedicated to probiotic foods. If your favourite shop doesn't carry them, you can ask the manager to order some for you.

Unfortunately, probiotic foods can be pricey—for example, a jar of probiotic sauerkraut can cost a lot more than a can of the non-probiotic hotdog topping. My hope is that as these foods become more popular, their prices will come down, which is already happening in some markets.

In this chapter, I'll introduce you to some of these probiotic foods, and offer you tips about what to look for and what to avoid. I'll also share ideas about how to include them in your diet.

Yogurt

In the US, yogurt is the mother of all probiotic foods and the one type of living food you may already have in your kitchen. Yogurt is made by adding live bacteria to milk from a cow, goat, or sheep, or to soya milk. It is believed to have originated in Turkey, but most countries that kept animals for milk had some kind of yogurt-like food—in some places, yogurt has been made with the milk of yaks, camels, or even horses.

Plain yogurt tastes tart, tangy, and creamy. For people who aren't accustomed to eating yogurt the flavour can be a little too tangy, but believe me, your taste buds will adjust and you'll find yourself enjoying the flavour before you know it once you mix in some other gut-friendly ingredients.

Yogurt comes in full-fat, low-fat, and nonfat versions. I like the flavour of full-fat yogurt, and there's some research that suggests the fat in full-fat grass-fed yogurt may actually be best for us. In general, I recommend full-fat dairy products such as yogurt, kefir, milk, and cheese. I know this sounds paradoxical, because for so long we've thought that nonfat dairy is the best choice, especially for weight loss. But the research isn't backing this up. In fact, I keep reading more data about full-fat dairy being associated with weight loss, not gain, as well as lower diabetes risk. I don't think we can ignore these findings. For this reason, I recommend full-fat organic dairy (or low fat if you prefer the taste) rather than nonfat dairy/skimmed milk.

The most important thing I recommend, though, is paying close attention to the flavouring because most yogurt does have added sugars—usually in the form of vanilla or fruit flavour. It's amazing how much sugar and empty calories these flavourings can bring to a serving—anywhere from 50 to 75 calories or more. I highly recommend that you skip all those sugary flavours and go with plain and add fresh fruit instead. If you enjoy the jelly-like fruit in flavoured yogurts, try mashing berries or soft fruit and add them to plain yogurt. I also like adding spices such as cinnamon and nutmeg to my yogurt. If you really can't stand plain yogurt, stir in a teaspoon of honey or maple syrup. (I confess to not loving the taste of plain yogurt so that's what I do.) But over time I've added less and less as my taste buds have adjusted to the tangy flavour.

The best part about yogurt is that it can fill in for milk, cream, buttermilk, and other dairy foods in smoothies, salad dressings, and breakfast granolas and porridges. It's delicious mixed with fresh fruits, nuts, granola or toasted oats, and spices such as cinnamon. It's also a great base for dips that make raw fruits and vegetables more enjoyable to eat. And if you like creamy, mayonnaise-based salad dressings, swap in plain yogurt instead of mayo, add in some extra herbs, spices, and garlic, and you'll have a delicious dressing that's far healthier for you than those heavy mayo dressings.

Here's good news if you're lactose-intolerant: many people who get bloating, wind, or other symptoms when they drink milk are able to digest yogurt because bacteria in yogurt help digest the lactose (milk sugar) that can cause discomfort.

Yogurt Buying Guide

- ▶ To make sure the yogurt you're eating contains living bacteria, look for the words "live and active cultures" on the label. This is important—not all yogurt has living bacteria in it.

- ▶ Different brands of yogurt may contain different strains of bacteria, so you may want to stock up on a few different brands. My favourite yogurt isn't organic but it is made with milk from grass-fed cows raised without the use of recombinant bovine growth hormone (rBGH), and it contains no gelatins or gums.

▸ So many yogurts contain sugar, artificial colours, artificial flavours, and even chopped-up cookies and candy pieces. You know you shouldn't buy these for yourself, and I hope you won't buy them for your kids, either. Instead, bring your kids up eating real yogurt flavoured with fresh fruit rather than artificial flavours, added sugar, and other junk ingredients.

▸ Many yogurts contain gums, gelatins, or other thickeners. Avoid these if you can, and go with more natural brands if they're available. Why eat gums when you can have yogurt that's thickened naturally by billions of Little Buddies?

▸ Yogurt comes in several forms—ordinary yogurt, Greek yogurt (which is thicker, more tart, and contains more protein and fewer carbohydrates), and "drinkable" yogurt, which you can drink right from the bottle, mix into smoothies, or pour over cereal, granola, or fruit. Be careful buying drinkable yogurt—a few brands are healthy choices, but many are loaded with artificial crap, so be sure to read labels carefully.

▸ Although frozen yogurt is an enjoyable treat, don't eat it if you're looking for a probiotic food. Few or no living bacteria are found in commercially made fro-yo. That also goes for yogurt-covered raisins, yogurt-covered pretzels, and other confections, as well as the yogurt coating on some energy bars.

Kefir

Truth be told, when I started writing this book, I didn't know much about kefir. Turns out it's a fermented milk drink made by adding a "fermentation starter" of yeast and bacteria to milk from a cow, goat, or sheep. Kefir is pronounced kuh-FEER, though you'll often hear it called KEE-fer. It is believed to have originated in the North Caucasus Mountains between Europe and Asia. I tried it for the first time this year and it tastes tangy and creamy, sometimes buttery or acidic, like buttermilk. Kefir is sometimes described as being a thinner version of yogurt.

What's cool about kefir is it tends to contain more strains of bacteria than yogurt. Like yogurt, kefir can take the place of other milk-like products. Use it on cold cereal instead of milk, in place of buttermilk or mayonnaise in salad dressings, poured over fresh berries instead of cream, and as a creamy ingredient in cold soup. It can also be used to marinate meat such as lamb or pork. Personally, I have started to use it instead of milk as a base for my smoothies since it adds a nice probiotic punch.

Kefir Buying Guide

► To make sure the kefir you buy contains living bacteria, look for the words "live and active cultures" on the label.

► Kefir comes in full-fat, low-fat, and nonfat versions. Calorie totals are similar to milk; if you're trying to lose weight, consider low-fat kefir to save calories. The brand I like has 90 calories in a one-cup serving of low-fat plain kefir, and 160 calories for full-fat.

► Kefir comes in plain and flavoured varieties; I recommend you stick with plain because flavouring adds anywhere from 40 to 60 or more calories per serving and around 18 or more grams of sugar, which your body and your Little Buddies simply don't need.

► Choose organic or conventional kefir; I usually buy organic to avoid pesticide residue and other chemicals that may be harmful to gut bacteria.

Kimchi

Kimchi, pronounced KIM-chee, is a traditional Korean dish of fermented vegetables. It's made with a wide range of veggies, such as daikon radishes, peppers, cabbage, spring onions, carrots, leeks, onions, cucumbers—you name it. And it usually contains ginger, garlic, spices, chilli pepper flakes, and other strong flavours. Traditionally, kimchi was stored in underground jars.

Kimchi is pungent and spicy, crunchy and earthy, bold and flavourful, and sometimes bubbly. It is the kind of food that fills your kitchen with its aroma the minute you open the jar. If you like the pickled ginger that's sometimes served with sushi or sashimi, you'll probably like kimchi. I can't lie: I don't like kimchi. It's a little bold for me but you won't know for yourself unless you try it!

Traditionally, kimchi is a side dish served at almost every Korean meal. It can be eaten as is or with rice, pasta, whole grains, meat, fish, other vegetables, or beans. It also gives a jolt of flavour to burritos, salads, veggie burgers, and sandwiches. You can add it to lunch bowls or dinner bowls for a dose of flavour and crunch.

Kimchi Buying Guide

- ▸ To make sure the kimchi you buy contains living bacteria, look for the words "live and active cultures" or "live enzymes" on the label.

- ▸ Some brands contain a lot of salt; check the label for sodium content.

- ▸ Some brands contain sugar; a little is okay, but avoid brands with lots of added sugar. Some contain no added sugar and are vegan-friendly and gluten-free.

- ▸ Kimchi also shows up in other foods; for example, I've seen kimchi drinks. Before you buy these, check the label to make sure they contain live, active cultures and no added sugar or artificial flavourings and an acceptable amount of sodium.

Live-Culture Sauerkraut

I should start by telling you that probiotic live-culture sauerkraut is *not* the canned stuff that you grew up eating on hotdogs. Yes, the sauerkraut from your childhood is indeed pickled cabbage, but the canning process kills any Little Buddies that may be present. Live-culture sauerkraut is made and packaged in a way that allows microbes to stay alive during the time the shredded cabbage ferments in brine. And it is made just with cabbage, salt, and water—not vinegar, which can kill microbes. I always thought of sauerkraut as being a European food, but it actually originated in China. I hated sauerkraut as a kid but I have learned to love it as an adult.

Savoury, crunchy, tart, and salty, this sauerkraut is better than any of the canned stuff. The brand I buy has a fresh, bracing taste that leaves canned sauerkraut in the dust. It's not widely available, but as the popularity of fermented sauerkraut grows, I'm sure more shops will start to carry it. Like kimchi, sauerkraut can go with almost anything—fish, meat, salads, lunch bowls, or dinner bowls. Mix it into veggie slaws or burritos for a burst of flavour.

Sauerkraut Buying Guide

▸ To make sure the sauerkraut you buy contains living bacteria, look for the words "live and active cultures" or "live enzymes" on the label.

▸ Flavoured sauerkraut may contain excessive salt or sugar, so be sure to check the nutrition labels.

▸ Vinegar kills beneficial bacteria, so live-culture sauerkraut won't have it. But the fermentation process creates a tart flavour that mimics that of vinegar.

▸ Cold helps keep the Little Buddies in sauerkraut alive, so look for probiotic sauerkraut in the refrigerator cases. You may also see probiotic pickles, which, like sauerkraut, are made without vinegar.

Kombucha

Kombucha (kom-BOO-cha) is a beverage made by adding yeast and bacteria to sweetened green or black tea and allowing it to ferment. (Sometimes fruit juice or other flavourings are added as well.) It is sometimes referred to as "mushroom tea" but it isn't made with mushrooms. It gets that name from a mushroom-shaped glob formed in the tea when culture ferments. Kombucha comes from China, where it has been consumed for centuries. Traditionally, it was thought of as an elixir of youth that had almost magical health benefits.

Kombucha can have a sweet/sour flavour with acidic, vinegar-like overtones. It may be a bit bubbly (almost like it's mildly carbonated) and can have a slightly alcoholic taste. Although it's called tea, it doesn't taste at all like your everyday cup of Lipton. Kombucha often has sediment in it, which are the remains of the Little Buddies that performed the fermentation work. It's perfectly fine for you but I admit, I don't like to think about that when I'm drinking it!

This is a beverage meant to be enjoyed cold and many people love its taste. I personally didn't fall in love immediately with the taste, but I do tend to keep a bottle in the fridge and drink it from time to time simply for the probiotic benefit.

Kombucha Buying Guide

▸ Because pasteurization (high heat) would kill the Little Buddies in kombucha, only unpasteurized (or raw) kombucha contains live, active cultures. Check the label.

▸ Because it is a fresh food, kombucha must be refrigerated.

▸ As kombucha becomes more popular it may be added to other beverages for marketing purposes. Be wary of these products, because they may contain few or no live and active cultures, and they may be high in sugar or calories.

▸ The fermentation process that turns tea into kombucha also creates alcohol—not much, but enough that it's a concern for recovering alcoholics, pregnant women, and other people who should or want to avoid alcohol completely.

Tempeh

Tempeh (TEM-pay) is fermented soybeans. It is made by adding a yeast-based starter culture (full of Little Buddies) to partially cooked, water-soaked soybeans; as the culture ferments, it transforms into a firm, cake-like food. Tempeh originated in Indonesia, where it is traditionally sold wrapped in banana leaves. Tempeh can also be made with other types of beans or a mixture of beans and grains.

Tempeh is another food that I had not tried until recently. It has a chewy, nutty, earthy, sometimes smoky taste. People who like mushrooms tend to enjoy the flavour of tempeh. It is a versatile food that can be used in many different ways, often in place of meaty protein foods. Although some people eat tempeh raw, more often it is cut into slices or chunks (as you would with boneless, skinless chicken breast meat) and stir-fried, baked, or steamed. It can be added to stir-fries, soups, chilli, salads, and stews.

Tempeh Buying Guide

▸ Pasteurization (processing with high heat) can kill the microbes in tempeh, so not all of the tempeh available contains live and active cultures. Be sure to check the label of the tempeh you're buying to be sure it contains living cultures.

- Tempeh with live cultures must be kept cool, so look for it in the supermarket refrigerator or freezer cases.

- Shop-bought tempeh may contain preservatives or additives; check the label.

- Look for tempeh in natural food stores, health food shops, and Asian markets.

- If possible, choose tempeh made from soybeans that are grown organically.

- The plant-based oestrogens in soya foods may help reduce menopausal hot flashes, but people with hormonal-linked cancers and health conditions are sometimes advised to limit soya intake. Check with your doctor if you have questions about eating soya foods.

- Tempeh can be made with wheat or barley, so if you're eating gluten-free, be sure to check labels or call the manufacturer to find out what's in their product.

Miso

Miso (ME-so) is a paste made when cooked soybeans, salt, and cooked grains (sometimes) are fermented with bacteria and mould and then aged for as long as three years. Traditionally, miso is a Japanese food.

Miso provides a salty, savoury flavour that can also be sweet or fruity. It can be eaten by stirring it into cold sauces, salad dressings, dips, vegetables, and other cool dishes. You've probably heard of hot miso soup, but adding it to hot soups kills the Little Buddies in it. So if all you're looking for is flavour it's fine to heat miso, but if you're looking to maximize the benefits to your gut bacteria and you're eating miso as a probiotic food, keep it cool.

Miso tends to be high in sodium. If your doctor has told you to watch your sodium intake, read the label and factor in the sodium content of miso when you decide whether and how much of it to eat.

Miso Buying Guide

- Because pasteurization (high heat) kills microbes, choose unpasteurized miso that is sold in jars in the refrigerator case.

- If possible, choose miso made from soybeans that are grown organically.

- Miso can be made with barley and other gluten-containing grains such as wheat, barley, or rye, so if you have coeliac disease or gluten sensitivity, choose miso made without gluten.

- As miso becomes more popular, it's being made with other kinds of pulses, such as chickpeas or aduki beans, in addition to or instead of soybeans.

Other Probiotic Foods

As word spreads about the benefits of supporting gut bacteria through diet, more and more probiotic foods will be appearing in shops. Some will be legit; others will probably have only a small amount of useless probiotics added simply for marketing purposes; many others will have probiotics on the ingredient list but will be processed in a way that kills any beneficial

Make Your Own Probiotic Foods

An alternative to buying probiotic foods—which can be expensive—is to make your own. This is a great option for people who enjoy spending time in the kitchen. However, when it comes to fermenting foods and working with live and active cultures, it's best to know what you're doing, or you run the risk of having unsafe microbes growing in your foods. Be sure to use only reputable fermentation guides, and follow recipes and directions carefully—the last thing you want is to develop a microbial-based illness or infection. Here are some books to help guide you:

- *Fermented Foods at Every Meal* by Hayley Barisa Ryczek (Fair Winds Press, 2016)

- *The Art of Fermentation* by Sandor Ellix Katz (Chelsea Green Publishing, 2012)

- *Fermented Vegetables* by Kirsten K. Shockey and Christopher Shockey (Storey Publishing, 2014)

- *The Big Book of Kombucha* by Hannah Crum and Alex LaGory (Storey Publishing, 2016) bacteria. That's what's happened with yogurt; some yogurt products don't contain any live and active cultures, but people don't necessarily realize that when they buy them.

A good rule of thumb is to read the label carefully and look for the words "live and active cultures" or "live enzymes."

Some foods, such as sourdough bread, start out containing living cultures. But the intense heat of the cooking process kills them. Or they can be killed by the pasteurization process, which is designed to eliminate bad bacteria but takes out anything in its path. Keep in mind that with foods such as yogurt and kefir, the milk they're made of is pasteurized before the addition of live, active cultures.

Other ingredients can harm the Little Buddies in food, too—vinegar being a great example. That's why sauerkraut or pickles made with vinegar don't contain live, active cultures.

Coming Up

Now that we've looked at all the different kinds of foods that are great for your gut, it's time to talk about some of the bacteria bullies that may be introduced to food during the growing process. In the next chapter, I'll share my thoughts and recommendations about choosing foods that are raised in the healthiest ways.

CHAPTER
11

Ban Bacteria Bullies in Food

Picture a beautiful summer tomato, with its smooth orange-red skin. It may have a stem and green leaves on top, or whitish-green pith where the tomato was attached to the plant on which it grew. Imagine cutting the tomato open and seeing its juicy red flesh and clumps of seeds. If you're a tomato lover, your mouth is probably watering at the thought of sinking your teeth into the delicious tomato you're seeing in your mind.

Unfortunately, what you *don't* see when you prepare and eat a fresh tomato or other produce are the pesticides and synthetic chemicals that may have been used to grow it. The same is true with a piece of beef, an egg, or a glass of milk. You see the food, but you don't see the chemicals, antibiotics, and potential toxins that were used to raise it. You don't know those things are there—but your gut bacteria do. These substances—or bacteria bullies, as I like to think of them—can cause serious harm to your Little Buddies. In fact, they're taking a big chunk of the blame for the damage being inflicted on the human microbiome in this country.

Unfortunately, we live in a world where most of our food is raised not by local farmers but by businesses that often care more about making money than providing us with the healthiest food. To maximize the bottom line, substances with uncertain impact on human health are often used. Our lawmakers allow this to happen, and consumers are left with a food supply full of potential toxins.

The chemicals and drugs in our foods can be hazardous for us and our Little Buddies. I'm not surprised that dramatic decreases in the vitality and health of the human microbiome coincide with huge increases in the uses of pesticides, antibiotics, and other chemicals in our agricultural system.

That's the bad news. The good news is that more and more people and businesses are realizing that banning bacteria bullies and eating pure food makes a lot more sense than eating food raised with potential toxins. More consumers are willing to pay for purely raised food, more farmers are committing to toxin-free growing, and more shops are carrying healthfully raised foods. We're even seeing some progress among giant agricultural businesses and fast-food chains that are answering their customers' demand for purer food by offering some alternatives to conventionally raised food.

In this chapter, we'll take a look at why eating purer foods matters to you and your Little Buddies. I'll share some tips to help you as you navigate your way through the shops. And, because pure food costs more than conventionally raised food, I'll help you decide how to prioritize your purchases to fit your budget.

We'll start with antibiotics. You know them as the medicines your doctor gives you when you're sick. But believe it or not, the majority of antibiotics in the United States are used on animals, not people—but we end up being affected by them anyway.

Antibiotics in Food

In chapter 12, I'll tell you all about how the antibiotics your doctor prescribes for you can impact your Little Buddies. But now that we're focused on food, let's look at antibiotics used in animals. Antibiotics were first developed in the late 1920s, and they became universally available in the US in the 1940s. They were considered a miracle drug for humans, because they cured a range of diseases that had previously killed millions of people.

After seeing how successful antibiotics were at treating people, veterinarians started using them to treat infected animals. But it took only a short time for farmers and big agricultural businesses to discover that antibiotics didn't just help sick animals—they helped healthy animals, too, by preventing certain diseases. And, as it turns out, they also helped animals gain weight faster.

This is good for farmers, who want to fatten up their animals and sell them at a high price. But many experts believe that the antibiotics that fatten up animals also fatten up the people who eat them. It's no surprise to me that the increase in antibiotic use in animals and the increase in human weight—the obesity epidemic—follow a similar upward trajectory.

Today, enormous amounts of antibiotics are routinely given to farm animals—in fact, some estimates are that 80 percent of the antibiotics made in the United States go to animals.

Antibiotic medications work by killing "bad" bacteria that can cause dangerous infections. But they also kill off good bacteria, like the Little Buddies in our guts and the guts of animals. What seemed like a good idea decades ago has grown into a problem that now threatens us all.

Antibiotic Resistance

Treating so many animals with antibiotics is contributing to the problem of antibiotic resistance throughout the world. Here's why: Antibiotics kill good bacteria as well as bad ones. When good bacteria die, bad bacteria can increase in number and strength. Eventually, bad bacteria can overcome an antibiotic's ability to kill or weaken them. This can lead to a problem known as "antibiotic resistance." When bacteria are antibiotic-resistant, it means that they need stronger and stronger antibiotics to kill them. And when bacteria become super-resistant—when they develop into the "superbugs" you may hear about in news reports—we run out of antibiotics that will eliminate them. This leaves patients in the very dangerous situation of bacterial infections that can't be treated or cured with the antibiotic drugs that currently exist.

Antibiotic resistance is a growing public health problem in the world today. When antibiotics don't work, the risk of serious illness and death from bacterial infection go up. According to the Centers for Disease Control and Prevention, two million Americans per year get serious bacterial infections that are resistant to antibiotics; 23,000 of those people die from those infections. Those numbers are expected to rise as antibiotic resistance gets worse, which it likely will unless we start making some serious changes.

Unfortunately, the overuse of antibiotics in farm animals is a big contributor to the development of antibiotic resistance. Administering antibiotics so routinely to so many animals helps create antibiotic-resistant superbugs.

Collateral Damage

Health experts and medical organizations are beginning to recognize how dangerous it is for us to be pumping our meat animals full of antibiotics. For example, the American Medical Association (AMA) has called for a reduction in the use of antibiotics in farm animals. The AMA is most concerned with antibiotic resistance. I'm worried about that, but I'm also very concerned about the effect that antibiotics in meat and poultry have on the human microbiome—as are many of the scientists who study gut microbes.

Research suggests that eating too much of the wrong kind of meat can have a detrimental effect on the health of our gut bacteria. But here's the thing: I don't think it's necessarily the meat that is causing problems for gut microbes. I think some of it has to do with the antibiotics that conventional animals are jacked up with. I bet that if studies were done on people who eat antibiotic-free meat, the findings might be a lot different.

For all these reasons, I recommend that when you eat meat, eggs, and other foods that come from animals, you choose foods from animals that are raised *without* any antibiotics. I know they're more expensive, but I think they're worth it and it may just save you money in the long run by lowering your healthcare expenses.

Many Benefits

When you buy organic meats, eggs, and dairy products, you're also protecting yourself from the growth hormones that are often used in conventionally raised animal products. You also get better taste, in my opinion—I think organically raised meat, eggs, and dairy have a fresher, more enjoyable flavour than their conventionally raised counterparts.

One way to defray the higher cost of antibiotic-free meat is to eat less meat overall, and to rely more on plant proteins, such as beans, nuts, and seeds, in your diet. When you reduce your overall intake of meat, you can afford to pay more for higher-quality meat on the occasions when you do decide to have it.

Organic Grains

In addition to buying organic meat, poultry, and produce, you can also buy organic grains, such as rice, quinoa, breads, and crackers. Should you go organic in the grain aisle as well? And what about pulses? Is it worth it to buy organic beans, peas, and lentils? My answer to that question is yes, if you can afford it, since grains and pulses are plant foods treated with pesticides. But if your budget is tight, focus primarily on organic meat, eggs, and dairy foods. And when you buy organic meat, you protect yourself and your Little Buddies from antibiotics, too.

Think of it this way: if you spend £15 on antibiotic-free beef for tonight's dinner, you can even things out tomorrow night by spending just a few pounds on a meal of beans and brown rice with veggies or some other meatless meal. For the same amount of money, you can get two much higher-quality meals than you would if you bought conventionally raised beef two nights in a row.

I also recommend that you buy grass-fed meat. Grass-fed animals produce meat that is higher in nutrients than conventionally raised animals. Not all organic meat is grass-fed, and not all grass-fed meat is organic, so make sure to read labels before buying. Organically raised animals are not exposed to pesticides, hormones, antibiotics, or chemical fertilizers.

As for eggs, I suggest you buy organic eggs that are raised without hormones or added antibiotics, from hens fed vegetarian diets rich in omega-3 fatty acids. In my opinion, these eggs really are much better for you and your gut than factory-raised conventional eggs. And I think they taste better, too! If you're lucky enough to live near a farm that raises organic eggs, definitely give them a try—they are absolutely delicious.

I'm not saying you have to buy organic, antibiotic-free animal foods exclusively. But I think of it this way: Every conventionally raised hamburger, chicken breast, or egg you eat adds to your body's antibiotic load, increasing the bacteria bullies in your system. By eliminating as many of those bullies as possible, you give the beneficial bacteria in your body a little extra help. If your goal, like mine, is to help your Little Buddies as much as possible, buying antibiotic-free animal foods makes a lot of sense.

Dr. T's Quick-Prep Tip

To make an amazing burrito in one minute, do this: Spoon black beans straight from the can onto a whole-grain tortilla and sprinkle with grated cheese. Slip it into the microwave and heat until the cheese melts. Then add guacamole or avocado and salsa or hot sauce, and you're ready to eat!

And for veggie nachos that are ready in a split second, sprinkle black or pinto beans straight from the can onto whole-grain crisps. Top with grated cheese, salsa, guacamole, and a dollop of Greek yogurt. Voila—nachos!

Pesticides in Produce

Anyone who's ever grown vegetables or flowers knows how frustrating it can be to look in the garden and see that your green beans or your roses have been nibbled half to death by bugs or some other kind of pest. When this happens, the solution is often to spray those plants or the soil they grow in with chemicals that repel or kill pests, weeds, or fungus. I get it: when you work hard to grow something, and a pest is wreaking havoc, it's a natural inclination to grab a spray that protects your plants, not thinking that it might be toxic.

The downside of many pesticides is that they contain chemicals that have been linked to cancer, disruption of hormones, and other serious health problems. And although we don't know the full extent of their impact on gut bacteria, it certainly makes sense that chemicals designed to kill pests would also harm or kill our Little Buddies.

Unfortunately, conventionally grown fruits and vegetables are raised with large amounts of pesticides. Although there hasn't been an enormous amount of research on this yet, I believe that future studies will find connections between pesticide use and damage to gut microbes.

When pesticides are used on produce, residue from those chemicals remains in and on the food. Peeling and washing fruits and veggies does remove some of the pesticide residue, but much of it remains. The best way to avoid pesticide residue is to buy organically grown fruits and vegetables.

Listen, I know that organic food is expensive. Luckily, as consumer demand has increased, prices have improved. I know it's unrealistic for most of us to switch completely to organic produce. But if you can swing it financially, I recommend it, especially for fruits and vegetables you eat frequently and where you don't peel off the skin.

If you can't afford any organic produce, don't let it stop you from eating fruits and vegetables. Eating conventionally grown produce is far better than eating no fresh produce at all.

Save at the Shops

One way to save money is to buy frozen organic fruit, which can be a lot cheaper than fresh—and it lasts longer, so you won't end up wasting any. My freezer is always full of bags of frozen organic raspberries, blueberries, and mixed berries.

If you're lucky enough to have a garden and to live somewhere with a good growing season, you can grow some of your own produce. There are lots of natural ways to protect your garden from pests without using pesticides—for example, a mild soap-and-water solution can ward off some pests. And planting certain flowers in your garden can attract bugs who feast on annoying pests. To learn more, check out websites and books on organic gardening.

Another option is to use the Environmental Working Group's list of the "cleanest" and "dirtiest" produce—those with the least and most residual pesticides—to make your buying choices. Here are the latest recommendations from the EWG, with "the Dirty Dozen" being the ones you should make the greatest effort to buy organic:

- ▶ **The Clean 15:** Avocados, sweetcorn, pineapples, cabbage, peas (frozen), onions, asparagus, mangoes, papayas, kiwi, aubergines, honeydew melon, grapefruit, cantaloupe, cauliflower.

- ▶ **The Dirty Dozen:** Strawberries, apples, nectarines, peaches, celery, grapes, cherries, spinach, tomatoes, peppers, cherry tomatoes, and cucumbers.

And remember, you don't have to take an all-at-once approach to eating purer food—I'm not suggesting that you switch from a 100 percent conventionally raised diet to a 100 percent organically raised diet. Start with the items you and your family eat most often—maybe it's yogurt, eggs, apples, and berries—and add more as you go along. As you transition to foods that are raised more purely, you should be steadily improving the environment in which your gut bacteria live, and the global environment in which we all live.

Coming Up

Eating fantastically fabulous high-fibre food is a huge win for your Little Buddies. But there's even more that you can do for them. In the next section of the book, we'll look at all of the other steps you can take to protect, support, and increase your beneficial bacteria.

PART
III

Other Ways to Boost Gut Health

Improving your diet is one extremely important way to foster the health and well-being of the Little Buddies who do so much for you. But it doesn't stop with food. There are plenty of other important steps you can take to protect and support the beneficial inhabitants of your belly's microbe community. That's what we'll cover in this part of *The Lose Your Belly Diet*. I'll tell you some of the important things that you can do—as well as things you can avoid—to be your Buddies' best friend.

CHAPTER
12

Avoid Unnecessary Antibiotics

It's time to talk about one of the biggest threats to our Little Buddies: unnecessary antibiotics.

Like most people, you've probably taken antibiotic medications. These drugs work by killing or weakening bacteria that cause dangerous infections. Antibiotics, which, as I mentioned, were first discovered in the 1920s and became universally available in the 1940s, changed the world by offering cures to many infectious diseases that had previously been incurable.

One of those diseases is tuberculosis, a potentially deadly bacterial lung infection. Before antibiotics were discovered, doctors had no cure for tuberculosis, and many of the people who got it died. When antibiotics became widely available, deaths from tuberculosis, or "consumption" as it was often called, fell rapidly.

Antibiotics are one of the most important medical discoveries in the twentieth century, having saved an estimated 200 million lives worldwide. But antibiotics also have a dark side. Yes, they are remarkably effective at killing *dangerous* bacteria. But we now know that they are also remarkably effective at harming *good* bacteria. And because of this, antibiotics—the miracle drugs that saved millions of lives—now pose a big threat to human health, in part because of their impact on the human microbiome.

Don't get me wrong: I'm not saying we should never use antibiotics. The truth is, they do save lives, and there are many situations in which prescribing an antibiotic is the very best choice for health and life. When I talk about antibiotics being a threat, I'm referring to situations in which they are used incorrectly, or when they are overused—times when healthcare providers prescribe a course of antibiotics when the better choice would be just to sit back and give the body time to heal itself.

But the fact is, antibiotics are tremendously overused, and this overuse is wreaking havoc on good bacteria while causing dangerous bacteria to mutate and become even more dangerous. And so, as we talk about taking steps to protect, support, and increase the beneficial bacteria in our own personal microbiome, we really do have to look at the overuse of antibiotics by individuals and as a society. While acknowledging the value of these medications, we also have to recognize their risks. The miracle drugs that have saved so many lives are also harming us.

It all sounds kind of scary, I know. But I'm not telling you all this to frighten you. Instead, I want to empower you. An important way to help protect your Little Buddies is to take antibiotics only when they are completely necessary—when the advantages outweigh the risks. By understanding what antibiotics can and can't do, you can work with your healthcare providers to make the best decisions about using antibiotics in a way that will protect your health and the lives of your gut bacteria.

An Epidemic of Overprescription

Antibiotics make their way into the human microbiome in two ways: through drugs that we take directly, and through the antibiotics given to farm animals that we eat as food. We talked about antibiotics in food in chapter 11, so now we'll look at the antibiotics we take directly—the ones that are prescribed by our healthcare providers.

Antibiotics work by killing or disabling bad bacteria. But as I mentioned earlier, they also kill good bacteria. When researchers look at people's stool samples before and after a course of antibiotics, they see direct evidence of the toll antibiotics take on good bacteria. Large decreases in gut bacteria have been found after taking antibiotics, and the stronger the drug, the greater the damage to our good Little Buddies.

For example, exposure to amoxicillin taken by mouth has been found to cause a decrease in gut microbes that lasts for at least one to two months. Broader-spectrum antibiotics, which kill a wider variety of bacteria, are believed to cause even more long-term damage to beneficial gut microbes.

Antibiotics are among the most commonly prescribed drugs in America—especially azithromycin and amoxicillin. In one year, more than 262 million courses of antibiotics are prescribed in doctors' offices, clinics, and other out-patient settings. Think about it: that's the equivalent of giving an antibiotic prescription to 83 percent of the people in this country every year.

Now, think about this: of all those antibiotic prescriptions that people get from their doctors, one-third to one-half are *not* necessary. That's right: somewhere between 87 million and 131 million antibiotic prescriptions should never have been written, filled, or taken by patients.

Missing the Target

It sounds hard to believe, but most of the unnecessary antibiotics in the US are prescribed for colds, sore throats, bronchitis, sinus infections, and ear infections that are caused by viruses. The problem with this is that antibiotics don't work on viruses! Viral illnesses don't respond to antibiotics! And yet, even though we know that antibiotics can't treat colds and other illnesses caused by viruses, healthcare providers are writing millions of prescriptions for them anyway. *This* is antibiotic misuse, and it is completely unacceptable.

You're probably wondering why in the world healthcare providers give out all those unnecessary prescriptions. I wonder that, too. Part of the problem is that providers have been a little late to the party when it comes to learning about the negative impact of antibiotics on gut bacteria. Many of them were trained when conventional wisdom held that antibiotics should be given "just in case" and many providers have been slow to change their prescribing habits.

Patients need to take some responsibility, too—although not as much as healthcare providers. As an emergency department doctor, I feel like I've seen it a million times: people with viral illnesses (or parents whose kids have viral illnesses) beg and sometimes bully their healthcare providers to prescribe antibiotics. It can be tough to say no to these people, although I think that more and more providers are learning to do so.

Instead of automatically writing antibiotic prescriptions, providers need to educate their patients about the harm these drugs can do when prescribed unnecessarily. Unfortunately, when a busy provider knows there are dozens of sick people waiting to be seen, and a patient is demanding antibiotics, it's often easier just to write the prescription. Additionally, patient satisfaction scores often are lower for physicians who *don't* prescribe unnecessary antibiotics. People often feel they have received substandard care when they leave without a prescription. That's a sad state of affairs if you ask me.

The Right Time

There are many times when antibiotics are the best treatment choice. For example, when a patient tests positive for bacterial meningitis, antibiotics are absolutely necessary and should be started immediately. Without treatment, bacterial meningitis can lead to brain damage, hearing loss, and even death. And antibiotics are typically used to treat throat infections.

But there are many situations that are not so clear-cut. Take ear infections in children, for example. Not so long ago, the standard treatment for any kind of ear infection was a course of antibiotics. But when researchers started looking a little more closely at ear infections in children, they discovered that many ear infections actually go away on their own, without antibiotics. For example, a type of ear infection known as acute otitis media (AOM), which is very common in children, often tends to clear up on its own, without antibiotics.

Over the past few years, professional organizations have been encouraging paediatricians to hold off on prescribing antibiotics for AOM unless they really are necessary. Instead, they recommend giving kids over-the-counter pain relievers that help them feel more comfortable during the "watchful waiting" period. If the infection doesn't go away in a certain period of time, the parents and the doctor can reconsider whether antibiotics may be necessary. But in many cases, the infections will go away without any antibiotics.

Looking Forward

There are lots of heavy thoughts in this chapter. But the good news is that I think we've reached something of a turning point in the prescribing of unnecessary antibiotics. We still have a long way to go, but more healthcare providers and patients are learning about the damage that unnecessary antibiotics can do to people and their Little Buddies.

In the past few years, major health agencies and medical organizations have been working hard to educate patients and providers about the dangers of antibiotic misuse. In some places, the number of unnecessary antibiotic prescriptions is starting to level off or go down.

In the meantime, how can you avoid taking unnecessary antibiotics? Start by choosing a provider who shares your concern about this very important issue. Some healthcare providers are much more likely to prescribe antibiotics than others.

If your provider recommends an antibiotic for you or your child, ask if it really is necessary. Talk about whether it might be okay to follow a watchful waiting strategy to see if the infection will clear up on its own. The time to take an antibiotic is when the benefits of taking it outweigh the risks—in other words, when a bacterial infection won't go away on its own and poses a health risk to you if it isn't treated.

Once you and your provider agree that an antibiotic is the best choice, talk about which antibiotic will be prescribed. A broad-spectrum antibiotic kills a wider range of bacteria than a narrow-spectrum antibiotic. It's best for your Little Buddies to choose an antibiotic with the narrowest spectrum—one that will treat your infection while inflicting as little collateral damage on your beneficial bacteria as possible. Broad-spectrum antibiotics are the right choice for some situations, but often, a less powerful choice will do the job. There's no point in using a two-by-four to kill a mosquito when a flyswatter will work just as well.

And don't pressure your provider to prescribe an antibiotic. I'm sad to say that many of my colleagues in the medical world prescribe unnecessary antibiotics simply because their patients pressure them to do so. Maybe the saddest thing of all is that our healthcare system has been set up to make many people believe that every time they get a cold they need to see a healthcare provider. Yet, the only cure for the common cold is time and treating your body right by getting plenty of rest and eating well. All the antibiotics in the world won't cure a cold. In fact, by taking unnecessary antibiotics, you may actually end up getting sick more often, because of their potential to have a negative impact on your overall immunity. What may seem like a quick fix could just lead to more illness in the future—and more antibiotics, and more damage to your personal microbiome.

If you are diagnosed with a bacterial infection that requires antibiotics, you can take steps to help your personal microbiome stay strong while you're on them. Start by making sure you're eating probiotic-rich foods every day, such as yogurt, kefir, and kimchi. Take daily probiotic supplements if your doctor thinks you should. And continue eating the high-fibre foods that nourish your gut bacteria. Taking these precautions can help support your gut bacteria while the antibiotic is doing its work.

Antibiotics are a valuable tool for fighting disease when we use them responsibly. But when we misuse them and when we expose ourselves to them unnecessarily, we do a huge disservice to our health and our Little Buddies. I urge you to take this issue seriously and to reduce the antibiotics that you're exposed to, both by avoiding unnecessary prescriptions and choosing foods that are raised antibiotic-free. Protecting your Little Buddies in this way not only helps your immune system stay strong, but can help you slim down and lose your excess belly fat, too.

Coming Up

In the next chapter, I'll tell you about 10,000 ways you can help your Little Buddies every day. But don't worry—you'll need only one pair of trainers, not 100 trillion.

CHAPTER
13

Strengthen Your Buddies with Exercise

It's no secret that exercise is good for your health. We've known that for a long time. Countless studies have shown that exercise can help prevent heart disease, some kinds of cancer, type 2 diabetes, obesity, depression, and anxiety, to name a few. Even if you've been sedentary for years or even decades, starting to exercise can begin to improve your health almost immediately. I've said it before, and I'll say it again: exercise does so much for our health that if we could somehow put it in a pill, it would be considered the most amazing wonder drug of all time, and people would be begging their doctors to prescribe it.

We understand some of the ways that exercise improves health. For example, it reduces heart disease risk by strengthening your heart muscle and opening up your blood vessels. And it cuts diabetes risk by stabilizing blood sugar and improving your body's ability to use insulin. There are a load of other ways in which exercise tackles disease risk. I could go on about that for pages and pages, but I won't, because I have a feeling that as someone who's concerned about health, you're probably pretty familiar with that already (even if you haven't quite got into an everyday exercise habit).

But here's something you are unlikely to have heard about, because researchers are really just figuring it out lately: in addition to helping your body in numerous ways, exercise also seems to help your Little Buddies. That's right—studies are finding that when you walk, run, jog, swim, bike, or do other kinds of exercise, in addition to all the good things you're doing for your heart, lungs, and muscles, you're also helping to protect and support the microbes living in your body.

Let's take a look at how exercise benefits your personal microbiome. And let's talk about what kinds of exercise are best for you and your gut. Relax—you don't have to start running marathons or spending endless hours huffing and puffing at the gym. Being active in a way that benefits your entire body is easier than you may think.

Prevention Paths

How do we know exercise helps our gut microbes? Researchers got their first evidence supporting this from animal studies. For example, mice that exercise have been found to have more gut bacteria than those that don't. And mice that exercise experience less damage to their gut bacteria from poor diets than those that don't exercise.

But what about people? Well, researchers have found similar results in humans. For example, scientists in Europe found that athletes had a much greater diversity of microbial species in their guts than nonathletes. And researchers in the US have noticed, when they analyze the gut microbes of various volunteers, that people who exercise have a more diverse gut microbiome than those who don't exercise. Exercisers also tend to have more of the super-helpful bacteria that keep people healthy. For example, one study found that people who exercise had greater numbers of bacteria that can protect them from certain diseases, such as colon cancer. And another discovered that nonathletes who exercise three to five hours a week had extra-high levels of a type of bacteria that improve immune function.

How would exercise help increase the types and numbers of gut microbes? There are a few possible explanations. Researchers believe that exercise may impact the action of enzymes that play a part in how energy and fat are used by the body. Exercise also affects the body's production of bile acids, which not only help with digestion but also appear to support beneficial bacteria.

Regular, moderate exercise also lowers inflammation throughout the body, which seems to protect your Little Buddies. It can also reduce the body's production of stress hormones such as cortisol, which seem to have a negative effect on gut microbes when their levels are too high.

Researchers still have a lot of work to do to tease out exactly how exercise helps our beneficial bacteria. That will keep them busy for a long time—but luckily, we don't have to wait for their results to figure out what we should do. The prescription is very simple: start moving.

The Best Moves

Moderate exercise seems to be the best bet for your body and your gut. Exercising moderately means working hard enough to give your heart a workout, but not so hard that you can't catch your breath.

For example, moderate walking means walking about 4 miles per hour, moderate jogging is about 5.5 miles per hour, and moderate biking would be around 10 miles per hour. That's what moderate means for the average person, of course. If you're very athletic, you can probably walk, run, or bike faster. And if you're sedentary, those "moderate" rates may be vigorous for you. That's okay. It doesn't matter how fast you move, as long as you're doing something that makes your heart pump faster than it does when you're sitting at your desk checking out Facebook.

Walking is a fantastic activity, one that I recommend for just about everyone because it has so many benefits and so few downsides. In addition to helping your Little Buddies, walking can lower your blood pressure, improve your cholesterol levels, and lower your diabetes risk—in fact, walking is every bit as good as running in reducing your risk for stroke and heart disease.

Other than a good pair of shoes, walking requires no special equipment or expensive gym memberships. You can walk in the morning, midday, or evening, alone or with other people, outdoors in your neighbourhood, or indoors on a treadmill or track.

In addition to walking or other activities that get your heart rate up, I recommend strength training to exercise your muscles. Strength training boosts your metabolism and helps you burn fat, build muscle, and strengthen your bones. You don't have to join a gym to strength-train, although of course you're welcome to. You can strength-train at home with exercise resistance bands. I use these bands to work out both at home and on the road. Unless you are a bodybuilder, you don't need to lift heavy weights.

Exercise Recommendations

Aim for these exercise goals:

- ► 30 minutes per day of moderate-intensity aerobic activity, such as brisk walking, jogging, swimming, or cycling.
- ► Muscle-strengthening activities that work all major muscle groups (legs, hips, back, abdomen, chest, shoulders, and arms) twice per week.
- ► Extra activity whenever you can squeeze it in—gardening, dancing, bike riding with your kids, walking the dog, and so on.
- ► Getting up off your butt more often—for example, walking or riding a bike to run errands instead of driving, standing rather than sitting at your desk at work, or riding a stationary bike rather than lounging on the couch while watching TV or reading.

One Move at a Time

Don't worry—you don't have to jump right in and do a lot of vigorous exercise immediately. If you're completely sedentary, I don't expect you to go from no activity at all to working out for hours a day. Start where you're comfortable—even 5 or 10 minutes a day is better than nothing—and work up from there. And remember, before making significant changes in your fitness routine, check in with your healthcare provider, especially if you have any medical conditions.

And don't feel discouraged if you've never exercised before—it is never too late to start. Get this: Researchers in England who were tracking the health of 3,400 people ages 55 to 71 found that those who became active during the eight-year study period were three times more likely to age healthfully than those who were inactive. And those who stuck with their exercise programmes during the study were seven times more likely to avoid aging-related health problems such as depression and dementia.

Listen, I've seen octogenarians in nursing homes who were able to retire their walkers after taking up strength training. Not only do they become stronger, but they improve their balance. This is a huge payoff because a loss of balance contributes to falls, which are one of the most common causes of injury,

Mood Mover

People exercise for a lot of different reasons. Personally, the number one reason I am active is that it helps to boost my mood. When I feel a bit of melancholy coming on, I make it a habit to do something active, even if it just means taking a quick walk outside. It's remarkable how much better I feel afterwards.

There's a good explanation for this. When we exercise, our brains release neurochemicals such as endorphins that actually make us feel better and that soothe anxiety. Exercise also lowers our body's production of the stress hormones that can leave us feeling rattled.

Relieving stress through exercise is good for your mind and it's also good for your gut. If you've ever had a stomach ache or diarrhoea when you've felt nervous or upset, you know there's a connection between your emotions and your gut. That kind of stress seems to affect your gut bacteria, too. Research has found links between high stress levels and a reduction in microbe diversity—probably because an overabundance of stress hormones has the power to harm gut bacteria.

disability, and shortened lifespan in older people. It truly is never too late to launch a fitness programme.

Begin with walking, and add in other activities as your fitness and confidence levels grow. Then, when you're ready, mix in some muscle-strengthening exercises. If you're not sure what to do, sign up for a class or do one or two sessions with a trainer who can teach you how to strength-train safely. Choose activities that you enjoy—you're never going to stick with it if you try to do something you hate. Doing something you like turns exercise from a chore into a kind of play. And once you start feeling more fit, you'll enjoy activity even more. Go ahead—have fun!

Step by Step

Many people swear by wearing a pedometer or a fitness tracker that counts their steps throughout the day and tallies them on their computer or smartphone. When you wear a pedometer or fitness tracker, you can make a game out of hitting your step goal every day. And if you're the kind of person who likes quantifying your efforts, keeping track of your daily, weekly, and monthly steps can be a really fun motivator.

I suggest that you aim for at least 10,000 steps of walking per day. If you're sedentary, you don't have to pressure yourself to hit that goal right off the bat. Nothing discourages people from exercise more than setting an unrealistic goal, failing to meet it, and then feeling bad about themselves. It's much better to start where you are, and increase gradually over time.

Try wearing a pedometer or fitness tracker and doing a typical amount of activity for one day. See how many steps you take. This is your baseline step count. Don't be discouraged if it's a small number of steps—that's okay! You're just starting.

Let's say your baseline step count is 3,000 steps. Rather than deciding to make a dramatic jump to a goal of 10,000 steps daily, aim just to add 1,000 steps a day to your daily tally for one week, for a total of 4,000 steps a day. Then, the next week, raise your goal to 5,000 steps a day. Continue that way, and within a few weeks you'll be at your 10,000-step daily goal.

How can you add more steps to your day? One option is to schedule walks during the day—a half-hour walk before breakfast, for example, or a 45-minute walk after dinner. But remember, you don't always have to set aside big chunks of time for walking. You can accumulate steps throughout the day simply by adjusting some of your common routines. For example:

- ▸ Walk rather than sitting when waiting at airports or in medical offices.

- ▸ Take the stairs instead of the escalator or lift.

- ▸ Set an alarm on your phone and take a five-minute walk every hour.

- ▸ Walk instead of sitting when you're talking on the phone.

- ▸ Go for walks rather than sitting in a coffee shop or bar when hanging out with friends.

- ▸ Keep your eye on your numbers throughout the day, and if you see yourself falling behind, squeeze in steps wherever you can. Make it a fun game, and you'll meet your goals.

▸ Set goals for the week, month, or season. I know someone who gets through the winter doldrums by setting a goal of walking one million steps between the first and last day of winter. Even though she has lived in the snowy Northeast her whole life, she doesn't like winter, and without some kind of motivation she'd hibernate like a bear. But having that one million step goal gets her out walking almost every day.

You know yourself—figure out what motivates you, and you'll find ways to be active every day. Be creative, and you'll think of lots of other ways to increase your daily step count.

Coming Up

You've probably heard about probiotic supplements. You may even take them. But do they really help with gut health? Maybe yes, maybe no—the answer to that question isn't as clear as it seems. In the next chapter, we'll talk about what we know (and don't know) about probiotic supplements.

CHAPTER
14

Consider Probiotic Supplements

As we've learned more about how the microbes in our guts help us, there's been a ton of focus on probiotic dietary supplements. These are capsules packed with live bacteria that can be taken daily, like a multivitamin. When probiotic supplements were first introduced they generated a huge amount of excitement. In theory, they would help build up and maintain the microbe communities in our guts and help protect us from some of the health problems that are associated with a lack of gut bacteria diversity.

But that's not quite how it's turned out—so far, at least.

Believe me: I love the idea of being able to send microbe reinforcements into our guts on a regular basis. I'd be thrilled if we could dramatically improve our health simply by swallowing a probiotic supplement every day. But unfortunately, although they may indeed be beneficial in some ways, they have yet to live up to the lofty hype that surrounded them when they were introduced. Overall, most researchers who have studied the effectiveness of probiotic supplements on human health during the past decade or so have been decidedly underwhelmed by their findings.

Where does that leave you and me? Should you be taking probiotic supplements? Should I be taking them? Or should we all hold off on them until researchers figure out how to formulate more effective probiotic supplements? The answer to all of those questions is a resounding "maybe." I know—that's not a very helpful answer. But when it comes to probiotic supplements, there isn't a clear yes-or-no answer for everyone.

Before I give you my recommendations, let's look at these questions a little more closely. Having a clearer understanding of what we know about probiotic supplements can help you decide what's best for you. And at the end of the chapter, I'll tell you where I stand on this question myself, and whether I pop probiotic supplements on a daily basis. You might be surprised by my answer.

Waves of Reinforcements

The word "probiotic" means "for life." Probiotic supplements are designed to support the life and diversity of your gut microbe community by bringing in beneficial bacteria and yeasts to the gut.

The principle behind probiotic supplements makes sense. After you swallow them, the Little Buddies in them would pass through the stomach and settle in to the intestines, where they would start doing some of the beneficial work that good bacteria do, such as helping out with the body's immune response. They would prevent harmful bacteria (pathogens) from attaching to intestinal walls, and they'd help produce acids (lactic acid, for example) that would assist in inhibiting the growth of harmful bacteria. Like sending in a second shift to a factory, these extra Little Buddies would help with all the gastrointestinal jobs that need doing.

But we're not sure that's actually what happens with all of the microbes in probiotic supplements. We know that some of them make it to their destination—researchers have found them in stool samples. But when we look for the expected health benefits in people who take probiotic supplements, we don't necessarily find them.

In fact, the US Food and Drug Administration (FDA) has not approved probiotic supplements for the prevention or treatment of any health problem.

That doesn't mean probiotic supplements aren't helpful. In fact, some studies have found that they're effective in some situations. But other studies that look at these supplements have found no evidence that they're providing any benefit for people.

Difficult to Study

Part of the challenge of studying probiotic supplements is that different brands contain different strains of bacteria. The most common bacteria used in probiotics are from groups known as *Lactobacillus, Bifidobacterium, Saccharomyces, Streptococcus, Enterococcus,* and *Bacillus.* But each of these groups contains many kinds of bacteria that may have different jobs to play in human health. It's possible that probiotic supplements don't contain the right microbes for the jobs we're asking them to do.

Also, whether a certain probiotic helps in a specific situation may depend on what kinds of Little Buddies people already have in their guts. It's very possible that probiotic effects differ from person to person based on the kind of microbes that do and do not reside in their bodies already, and right now we don't know enough about the human microbiome to tease out this kind of information—yet. Think of it this way: If you sprinkle grass seed on bare dirt, it's likely that a lot of grass will grow. But if that grass seed lands on a green lawn, the new seeds may not be able to grow—they may just sit there until they're eaten by birds.

Another challenge comes from the fact that supplements, in general, are not regulated closely by the FDA. Because of this lack of regulation, the contents of probiotic supplements may not be consistent, which can throw off study results. This has been a big problem with various types of supplements, not just probiotics.

When researchers have taken a close look at what's inside some of the probiotic capsules in shops, they have found some disturbing surprises. Sure, some of the products contain exactly what their labels say. But an alarming number of probiotic supplements do *not* contain what their packages promise. Some have ingredients that are not on their labels. Others *don't* have ingredients that *are* listed on their labels. And others have different amounts of bacteria than their labels claim.

The fact that some probiotic supplements have been found to contain ingredients that are not listed on their labels can be a problem for people with allergies and intolerances. For example, one study analyzed probiotic supplements for the presence of gluten, a protein found in wheat and some other grains that can cause gastrointestinal symptoms for people with coeliac disease and gluten intolerance. The researchers found that half of the probiotic supplements that were labelled "gluten-free" actually contained detectable levels of gluten—a surefire sign that we can't always trust the labels on our supplements. What makes this news even more disheartening is the fact that people with coeliac disease are frequent users of probiotic supplements because many believe that probiotics may help with their coeliac symptoms, when in fact the tainted supplements may actually make symptoms worse.

Probiotic Positives

Despite the difficulty of studying the effectiveness of probiotic supplements, there are some health conditions that really do seem to be helped by taking them. The research lines up in favour of probiotics for the following:

Diarrhoea: The evidence is pretty strong that probiotics can help with some kinds of diarrhoea, such as traveller's diarrhoea, antibiotic-associated diarrhoea, and acute diarrhoea, which is the kind of diarrhoea you get when you come down with a sudden infection caused by bacteria, viruses, or parasites. For example, studies have found that probiotics can prevent up to 85 percent of cases of traveller's diarrhoea.

Irritable bowel syndrome (IBS): The research is mixed on probiotic treatment for IBS, which is a gastrointestinal condition that causes a cluster of symptoms such as abdominal pain, diarrhoea or constipation, wind, bloating, and fatigue. IBS is fairly common, afflicting 10 to 15 percent of adults in the US. However, although not everyone with IBS benefits from probiotics, in some people, they significantly decrease symptoms, especially when they are combined with the right kind of high-fibre diet. People suffering with IBS should work closely with their healthcare provider to find the right eating plan to minimize their symptoms.

Inflammatory bowel disease (IBD): IBD is an umbrella term for a group of diseases, including Crohn's disease and ulcerative colitis, that are caused by chronic inflammation in the bowel. As with IBS, probiotic study results have been mixed for people with IBD; they seem to help some people but not others. For example, one study found that certain probiotics were as effective as a prescription medication for helping people with ulcerative colitis stay in remission. But research has been less promising for other people with IBD.

Atopic eczema (AE): AE is a skin condition seen most often in infants. Once again, probiotic treatment seems to help in some cases and not others. In one study, pregnant women with a strong family history of AE took probiotics during pregnancy and breast-feeding; their babies had a significantly lower risk of developing AE. But other studies haven't shown such strong results.

Other health conditions: There's not much evidence so far that probiotic supplements help with non-gastrointestinal health problems, despite what you might have read while cruising around the Internet or reading labels in health food shops. Why not? Here's my take. I strongly believe that gut bacteria have a huge impact on our health, and as we discussed earlier in the book, there are many health conditions that are associated with a lack of diversity among gut bacteria. But I'm not sure that the probiotic supplements that are now available are delivering the gut reinforcements that are needed to have an impact on all those health problems. Maybe they don't provide the optimal mix of gut bacteria, or maybe there's something about the way they're made or processed by the body that is preventing them from being effective.

I'm very willing to bet that when we learn more about probiotics, we'll figure out ways to make supplements more effective not just for GI health problems, but for a wider range of conditions. This is definitely a situation where more research and development is needed.

On the Fence

So, should you take probiotic supplements? Or should you wait a few years and wait until more effective ones are developed? Here's where I stand on this:

Overall, I don't feel that there's enough evidence in favour of today's probiotics to recommend that everyone take them. And I feel very strongly that eating a high-fibre diet that feeds your gut bacteria, eating probiotic foods daily, and taking the other Buddy-boosting steps in this book are the best ways to protect, support, and grow your gut microbe community. But I also think it makes sense for some people to take them—and for others to avoid them.

Let's talk about safety first. If you are generally healthy, probiotics are probably safe for you. Some healthy people do experience side effects from probiotics, but they are usually mild digestive symptoms such as wind, constipation, hiccups, or nausea that eventually go away. So on the positive side, probiotics seem to have few or no side effects in healthy people.

But the story may change for people with health problems that weaken the immune system. In these groups, there have been reports of serious infections as a result of taking probiotic supplements. If you have underlying health problems, are critically ill, have a weakened immune system, or have had surgery, taking probiotic supplements may put you at risk for severe side effects, such as serious infections that your body can't fight off. Because of this you should absolutely talk with your doctor before taking probiotics or any other supplements.

The same is true with children, babies, and pregnant or breast-feeding women: they shouldn't take probiotic supplements (or any supplements, for that matter) unless they first confer with their doctors. We think of over-the-counter supplements and medications as being benign because they're sold without a prescription. But don't be fooled; over-the-counter supplements can cause serious problems, so be aware.

Bottom Line: Who Should Take Them?

Now that we've talked about safety of probiotic supplements, let's look at their effectiveness for people who can safely take them. Here's what I recommend:

If you have GI problems: Overall, the evidence for gastrointestinal conditions such as IBS, IBD, and diarrhoea looks strong enough that if you have any of them, you should absolutely have a chat with your doctor about taking probiotic supplements. Unless there's a reason not to try probiotics, you can go ahead and give them a whirl. Find a product you trust, follow the directions on the label, and try them for a few weeks. If one brand doesn't seem to help, you can try another, because different brands provide different bacterial mixtures.

If you have other health problems: If you have non-GI health problems that you've heard may benefit from probiotic use, check in with your doctor, and if there are no reasons to avoid the supplements, you can give them a try for a month or two. If you see any improvements, great, and if you don't, then you can revisit with your doctor and decide whether to continue taking them or try something different.

If your doctor prescribes an antibiotic: Start by questioning your doctor to make sure you really need an antibiotic, because these powerful drugs kill good bugs as well as the bad ones, as discussed in chapter 12. If an antibiotic is the best choice, it's probably a good idea to take a probiotic for at least 7 to 14 days or more. But clear it with your doctor first.

If you're healthy and travelling: Taking probiotics may save you from an annoying case of traveller's diarrhoea, so if you're making a trip—especially if you're going out of the country or to a place where water contamination is an issue—it definitely makes sense to start taking probiotic supplements for three weeks or so before you begin your trip and continue taking them until you come home healthy.

If you are at risk for certain health conditions: Having a healthy community of gut microbes is associated with a lower risk of some kinds of health issues, such as obesity, diabetes, depression, eczema, and rheumatoid arthritis. Even though there isn't much evidence that today's probiotic supplements can prevent these conditions, it's possible they may provide some benefit that hasn't yet shown up in the research. So if you're healthy but concerned about developing any of these conditions, taking probiotics might make sense.

If you're healthy and none of these situations apply to you: There doesn't seem to be any harm in taking probiotic supplements if you're otherwise healthy. But there also doesn't seem to be a really strong reason to take them, either—unless you eat a really poor, low-fibre diet, which I doubt you're doing after reading this book! So if you feel better popping probiotics go ahead, but if you don't, that's a reasonable choice, too. If you do take them, and you start developing side effects, you may want to stop taking them, or try switching brands.

My Probiotic Decision

Thankfully, I fall into the "healthy" category, with no GI problems. It's been years since I've taken an antibiotic, my risk for other health conditions is low, and I eat a very healthy, high-fibre diet. In other words, there's no overriding reason for me to take probiotic supplements, so I don't bother with them. For now, I focus on eating a variety of probiotic-rich foods just like I recommend in this book.

Despite that, I am hoping that as we learn more about the human microbiome, we'll figure out ways to make probiotic supplements more effective. I do believe they have great promise for the future. If we can figure out how to make them work for a wider range of health conditions, we really could be onto something amazing. I am more than open to the idea of a daily probiotic supplement and hope that in the near future we will have more research to guide this choice.

Here's something to remember as you make your own choice about probiotic supplements. No matter how effective they are, vibrant gut health will never come from taking a pill. It's primarily about eating a healthy diet and making all of the other smart choices that are part of *The Lose Your Belly Diet*.

Coming Up

We've talked about a lot of steps you can take to protect your Little Buddies. Next, we'll make it a family affair by looking at how you can support your children's beneficial microbes too.

CHAPTER
15

Protect and Support
Your Family's Buddies

You don't just owe it to yourself to protect and support your Little Buddies. You owe it to your family, too. When researchers analyze the gut microbes of family members, they tend to find similarities—both positive and negative. There are a few reasons for this. When you share a home with people, you share microbes. You breathe the same air, are exposed to the same dust, play with the same pets, and eat similar food. Sexual partners share body fluids. And mothers pass their Little Buddies on to their babies.

When I say that you owe it to your family to protect and support your beneficial bacteria, I'm thinking about some research that's been done with mice. In studies, adult mice pass their microbes on to their babies. When parent mice have diverse, healthy microbe communities, their babies tend to, also. But when parent mice have poor internal ecosystems, or dysbiosis, their babies often do as well.

We don't know everything about how microbe communities are inherited or passed along among family members. But two of the mechanisms are becoming clear: how we give birth and how we feed our babies. We'll take a look at those two things in this chapter. I'll tell you what we've discovered as well as the steps you can take to protect and support your children's personal microbiomes.

Delivering Mum's Microbes

Babies are first exposed to beneficial bacteria within their mother's bodies. Then, more exposure comes at birth—especially if they are born vaginally. When babies are delivered vaginally, they leave the uterus, move through the birth canal (the cervix, vagina, and vulva), and then emerge out into the world. As you know if you've ever given birth or watched someone else deliver a baby, the birth canal is a messy place. Babies born vaginally come out of the birth canal covered with a goopy mix of fluids and waxy gunk that contains blood, mucus, and—as researchers have discovered—a wonderful soup of beneficial bacteria. It is during a baby's messy trip through the birth canal that it becomes colonized with bacteria from vaginal fluids.

However, not all babies receive this bacterial baptism on their first day of life. Those born by Caesarean section, or C-section, don't slide through all those messy fluids in the birth canal. When a woman has a C-section, her doctor removes her baby through a cut in her abdomen and uterus. Because a C-section is a surgical procedure, it is performed under sterile conditions, and a baby doesn't come in contact with all those birth canal fluids.

C-sections are very common in the United States, and are currently used in one-third of deliveries. These surgical procedures can and do save the lives of women and babies who are experiencing complicated deliveries. However, women's health experts agree that too many C-sections are performed in the US. In fact, as many as half of all C-sections are considered unnecessary.

When babies are born by C-section, they miss an opportunity to be colonized with the Little Buddies in Mum's vaginal fluids. They do pick up microbes in other ways—when their parents and other people hold them, for example, and through their everyday interaction with the environment. But when researchers analyze the microbes found in and on babies, they find more microbial diversity and greater numbers of beneficial bacteria in vaginally born babies than on babies born via C-section.

This may help explain, in part, why babies born by C-section have higher rates of health conditions such as obesity, asthma, and type 1 diabetes. Without a full complement of beneficial bacteria provided by vaginal fluids, C-section babies seem to be at a disadvantage when it comes to long-term health problems.

And so, for all these reasons, I join the American Congress of Obstetricians and Gynecologists (ACOG) and other health organizations in urging women to have C-sections only when medically necessary.

Avoiding Unnecessary C-Sections

Some C-sections are absolutely necessary—for example, when a woman has certain problems with her placenta, or if a baby isn't getting enough oxygen during delivery. However, many of the babies born via C-section can be safely delivered by vaginal birth.

Let's stop here. If you're a woman, you're probably thinking to yourself, how the heck can I avoid having an unnecessary C-section? Isn't it up to my doctor to make that call? And shouldn't my doctor know whether it's necessary to do a C-section?

You're right—it is your doctor's call. But too many doctors and other health-care providers are influenced by a pro–C-section culture at their hospitals. That's why, in order to avoid unnecessary C-sections, one of the first steps you can take is to look at the C-section rates at the hospital in which you plan to give birth.

Some hospitals have very high C-section rates. A 2016 *Consumer Reports* analysis found C-section rates in individual hospitals ranging from 11 percent of births to 53 percent of births. It makes sense that some hospitals have higher C-section rates—for example, those that handle a lot of high-risk deliveries. But even taking those into account, many hospitals still have a C-section rate that is too high. Some hospitals have a medical culture that pushes women to have unnecessary C-sections. C-sections are faster than vaginal births—as any woman who's been in labour for 20 hours can attest—and some hospitals prefer to get women in and out fast. So before you give birth, research your hospital's C-section rates, and if they're extremely high without explanation, consider another hospital.

Another way to avoid unnecessary C-sections is to talk with your health-care provider. Let your provider know that having a vaginal birth is important to you. If your provider belittles your wishes to give birth vaginally, consider seeing a different provider. You can also consider using a certified nurse-midwife or doula. Having continuous support while you're in labour can make it easier to cope with the challenges of a vaginal birth.

You can also educate yourself before delivery. Taking a childbirth class will help prepare you for birth and teach you strategies that will help you stay strong during labour. And take good care of yourself while you're pregnant. Gain the recommended amount of weight during pregnancy, exercise moderately throughout pregnancy, and see your healthcare provider regularly for prenatal checkups. Having good prenatal care helps lower the risks of developing complications that can require a C-section.

And there's one more thing. Remember that no matter how hard you try to avoid a C-section, it's not all in your control. Sometimes a C-section is necessary, no matter how carefully you try to avoid one. If you and your doctor decide that a C-section is the safest way to go, be okay with it. Having a healthy baby and safe delivery is your most important priority.

Buddies for Babies

Help may be on the way for babies born via C-section. Researchers are experimenting with a procedure called "microbial transfer." Using this procedure, bacteria-rich fluid from the mother's vagina is swabbed on her baby after C-section delivery in order to colonize the child with beneficial microbes.

Here's how researchers performed microbial transfer in a recent study done with four babies. Just before the mothers underwent C-section surgery, researchers used a piece of sterile gauze to collect some of the microbe-rich secretions from their vaginas. After the babies were born, they swabbed the babies' bodies (lips, faces, trunks, genitals, legs, arms, anuses, and backs) with the microbe-carrying gauze—which took about 15 seconds. Although the C-section babies weren't exposed to as much of their mother's fluids as babies delivered vaginally, the researchers hoped the swab would be enough to provide a bacterial baptism.

After one month, the researchers analyzed the bacteria in the swabbed babies' skin, gut, mouth, and anus. They compared it with the amount and types of bacteria collected from babies born by C-section who were not swabbed. The researchers found that swabbed babies had bacterial profiles that were similar to those of same-age babies born vaginally, which gave the researchers reason to believe that microbial swabbing may help C-section babies long-term.

More research is needed before microbial transfer becomes commonplace for women having C-sections—for now, the procedure is not widely available in hospitals. And follow-up studies will have to determine whether swabbed babies' rates of long-term health conditions are similar to that of babies born vaginally.

Researchers must also make sure that microbial transfer doesn't expose babies to microbes that could cause dangerous infections. Approximately 30 percent of women carry bacteria known as group B streptococcus, which can lead to meningitis and potentially fatal infections. And some women have sexually transmitted infections that could cause death or disability in newborns—we don't want to be swabbing babies with *those* bugs.

We obviously still have a lot to learn before we start using microbial transfers for every baby born via C-section. But in the meantime, it's good to know that at some point in the not-too-distant future, we may be able to give C-section babies the same bacterial advantages of babies born vaginally.

Microbe-Rich Food for Babies

Another bacterial baptism occurs after birth, when a baby begins breastfeeding. Breast milk is considered the perfect food for babies. Not only does it contain all the protein, fat, carbohydrates, and other nutrients a baby needs, but it delivers antibodies and hormones that help a baby grow and stay healthy. But there's more to breast milk than we previously realized. Although breast milk was once thought to be sterile, researchers have discovered that it also contains a rich variety of beneficial microbes that go directly from a mother's body to her baby's gut. When a mother breast-feeds, she's passing along her own beneficial microbes from her body to her baby's.

Here's something about breast-feeding that astonished me when I learned it: one of the components of human breast milk, a group of complex carbohydrates known as oligosaccharides, can't actually be digested by babies, because they don't have the enzymes needed to break them down. But researchers believe that the reason oligosaccharides are in breast milk is not to feed babies, but to feed their gut bacteria!

I wasn't at all surprised when I learned that breast-feeding helps pump up a baby's personal microbiome. We've known for years that breast-feeding provides babies with a kind of long-term health protection. Compared with formula-fed babies, babies who breast-feed have a lower risk of a long list of health problems, including asthma, childhood obesity, childhood leukemia, ear infections, eczema, diarrhoea and vomiting, lower respiratory infections, sudden infant death syndrome, and type 2 diabetes. Previously we assumed that the nutrients, antibodies, and hormones in breast milk were responsible for delivering all of those health advantages. But now it seems very likely that microbes play a big part as well.

As we learn more about the benefits of breast milk for babies, more women are choosing to breast-feed. Back when I was a baby, many mothers opted not to breast-feed because their doctors believed formula was better for babies than breast milk. I know, it sounds crazy, but a few decades ago, breast-feeding was thought of as low-class and old-fashioned, something done only by women who couldn't afford to buy formula. Now, of course, we realize that breast milk truly is the best food for babies, and about 79 percent of babies start off breast-feeding.

In order to give your baby the full benefit of breast-feeding, ACOG and other infant health advocates recommend that women breast-feed exclusively (or bottle-feed pumped breast milk) for the first six months of a baby's life, and continue breast-feeding while solid foods are introduced.

I understand that not all women can breast-feed for a full year, or even for six months—it's a lot to ask, and some women are simply unable for medical reasons. But as a doctor and as someone who's so committed to protecting, supporting, and growing our Little Buddies, I hope as a society we evolve to make breast-feeding as easy as possible for new mothers.

Even for those who can't breast-feed for a full six months or year, if they can do it for at least a few months. Or a few weeks. Or even a few days. It all helps.

If you feed your baby formula, you may notice that some brands contain probiotics. Although probiotic formulas seem safe for babies, there's no solid evidence that they provide babies with any long-term health benefits. Perhaps as researchers learn more about the strategic use of probiotic supplements, they'll figure out effective ways to add probiotics to formula.

Dump the Guilt

If you gave birth by C-section, or if you chose to feed your baby formula, you may be feeling unsettled thinking your baby's personal microbiome may not be as healthy as it could be as a result of those situations. Before you start feeling guilty, I want to remind you that we don't make health decisions in a vacuum.

When a woman is having a baby, doctors make delivery decisions based on a range of factors, the most important of which is to have a safe delivery. The same kind of thinking holds true for breast-feeding—it's optimal to breast-feed, but it's not possible for some women, and it's not the best decision for every woman and every family. That's okay. Instead of wasting energy on guilt, focus on providing your children with Buddy-friendly foods and an active lifestyle that will support their health for the rest of their lives.

And if it was you who was born via C-section or formula-fed, don't worry. It in no way means you can't live an incredibly healthy life. It is just even more incentive to focus on living a life that supports your Little Buddies.

Throughout Life

Once you start feeding your baby whole foods, you have an amazing opportunity to protect, support, and grow your baby's Little Buddies by serving super-healthy foods like the ones we've talked about in this book. You should always follow your paediatrician's advice on when to introduce foods and what is best for your child. But with the blessing of your doctor, offer your baby a wide range of microbe-supporting fruits, vegetables, pulses, and grains. And don't forget yogurt—babies love it!

In many ways the best thing you can do as your child grows is to set a great example: when you eat foods that nurture your Little Buddies as well as your overall health, your kids are watching.

Coming Up

The next Buddy-boosting step is one of the easiest of all. In fact, it might even save you some time with your housework!

CHAPTER
16

Get Dirtier

We've talked about lots of ways that you can protect, support, and increase the beneficial microbes in your own personal microbiome, from eating more fibre to avoiding unnecessary antibiotics. Now let's look at one more thing you can do—something that's actually pretty easy. Believe it or not, I'm recommending that you worry a little less about germs, especially in your own home and garden. Sometimes it's okay to get dirty!

We Americans live super-clean lives. We jump in the shower daily, wash our hands with antibacterial soaps frequently, and slather on hand sanitizers throughout the day. In our homes, we have cabinets full of powerful chemical cleansers that kill germs with a squirt and a wipe. Unfortunately, all of that washing and cleaning can have a negative impact on the Little Buddies in our personal microbiome. When we take steps to wipe away *bad* germs, we also end up killing *good* ones. We also encourage the *bad* germs to mutate and potentially become even more dangerous.

That's why I agree with the many gut researchers out there who are encouraging us not to worry quite so much about dirt and germs, and to let ourselves and our kids get dirtier.

Make no mistake: I'm not saying that we should stop washing our hands or start exposing ourselves to harmful germs. It makes total sense to keep things sterile in hospitals and to wash your hands after using the bathroom, when you're around sick people, and before and after handling food that could harbour pathogens that can cause food-borne illness. During cold and flu season, it makes perfect sense to use alcohol-based hand sanitizers when you're out in public—I can tell you, my hand sanitizer is never far away when I'm in airports and at public events where I meet a lot of strangers and shake a lot of hands. And pregnant women should exercise extra caution, because infections from germs in contaminated food and soil can cause pregnancy complications and raise the risk of some kinds of birth defects.

But there definitely are times when we can worry less about cleanliness and embrace the dirt, so to speak—times that you can set aside the hand sanitizers and high-powered cleaners. As you dig in your garden, play with your dog or cat, and hang out in your home, focusing less on killing germs may actually increase the beneficial microbes in your body. It also allows your immune system to get stronger.

A World of Dirt

Let's start with the great outdoors. When I was a kid growing up in the Midwest, I spent a huge amount of time outside playing. I also spent a lot of time exploring the family farm in Nebraska, and other than washing hands before dinner, nobody worried too much about all the dirt with which we came in contact on a regular basis.

Although I didn't know it at the time, my interaction with soil and animals during my childhood probably helped build up my gut microbes and my overall health, because it exposed me to a great diversity of microbes that made their way into my gut. In fact, research shows that kids who grow up on farms have lower rates of asthma and allergy—something that scientists refer to as "the farm effect."

One study looked at allergy and asthma rates in Amish children raised on farms in Indiana. The study found that only 5 percent of the children had asthma (compared with 11 percent of non-farm children) and 7 percent had allergies (compared with 44 percent of non-farm children). That's a pretty dramatic difference. Researchers believe that the farm effect is due to exposure to the high diversity of microbes on farms. Kids who are raised on farms pick up a wide variety of microbes as they interact with animals (and, to be honest, their poop), drink fresh unpasteurized milk, and come in daily contact with microbe-rich soil. These microbes take up residence in their guts and help diversify their personal microbiome.

Another study found that exposing mice to Amish farm dust over the course of a month helped protect them from reacting to allergens later, leading researchers to speculate that perhaps someday, human children could be partially inoculated against asthma and allergies with Amish dust. I know it sounds far-fetched, but it's certainly a worthwhile concept for researchers to consider.

This brings us around to something called the "hygiene hypothesis." According to this scientific theory, as societies' exposure to dirt and germs has gone down—as ours has in most of the US—the incidence of allergic and autoimmune diseases has gone up. Animal studies back this up: animals raised in sterile, bacteria-free conditions have been found to have weaker immune systems than those raised in ordinary situations.

We don't fully understand the connections between hygiene and disease. And we know that there are many kinds of diseases that occur far less often when a society has clean water and modern sanitation. But we also know that as societies get cleaner, the people who live in them are more likely to develop allergic and autoimmune diseases. It happened in the West, and it's happening in developing countries as they start to adopt Western ideals about cleanliness.

Why would better hygiene raise the risk of certain diseases? Here's what scientists think: Coming in contact with dirt and germs on a regular basis actually seems to help our immune systems get stronger and do their jobs more effectively. This seems counterintuitive—you might think that by protecting ourselves from germs we're helping our immune system. But the opposite seems to be true. The immune system actually seems to perform *better* if it has a chance to fight invasive microbes on a regular basis. Keeping active allows it to stay strong enough to do battle against more serious bacteria and viruses when they come along. Think of your immune system as a fire department that practises putting out small fires so that it's in great shape when a big fire breaks out.

When the world around you is super clean and your immune system doesn't have small fires to put out, it may start overreacting to harmless things such as pollen and foods, treating them as threats to your health and responding to them with an unnecessary immune attack. This raises your risk of immune-related conditions such as asthma and allergies. Your underused immune system may even attack your own body, which is what happens with autoimmune diseases such as rheumatoid arthritis, lupus, coeliac disease, and multiple sclerosis—diseases whose prevalence has been going up during the past decades.

I think this quote from William Parker at Duke University says it all: "The immune system is like a bored teenager. If you don't give it something to do, it will find something stupid to do."

A Dirtier Life

How can we get more dirt in our lives? We can't all pack up and move to farms, but we can take a few simple steps that will increase our likelihood of running into some helpful germs in our everyday lives.

Start by relaxing your home cleaning standards a bit. If you're someone who attacks every speck of dust or dirt with a bottle of powerful cleanser, hold back a little on that approach. The dust in homes can contain helpful microbes that can enter our bodies. And the chemicals in harsh cleaners, such as ammonia and chlorine, kill the good bacteria as well as the bad and can be harmful in other ways. Some dust and dirt in the house is okay. Don't bother with the white-glove test! And when you do clean, try to use natural cleaners or a cloth dampened with water or mild soap rather than an industrial-strength cleaner.

Hand washing is important, especially when someone in the house is sick. But there's no need to use antimicrobial cleansers or alcohol-based hand sanitizers on a regular basis. Plain-old soap and water work just fine. I personally use naturally derived foaming hand wash when I'm at home. Save the alcohol-based hand sanitizers for cold and flu season or when travelling.

I'm also inclined to suggest being a little less worried about babies and kids getting dirty. I'm not sure I agree with the gut researcher who suggested that we let our kids lick subway poles. But I do think that it's good for healthy kids to play and explore and interact with their environment—no need for parents to follow them around with a bottle of hand sanitizer. Check with their pediatrician first, of course, but unless there is some reason not to, go ahead and let kids make mud pies, dig in the garden, and pet animals in your neighbourhood and at petting zoos and farms. Exposure to the dirt and germs of everyday life can help strengthen their immune systems.

You may also want to think about getting a dog, if you don't already have one. Studies have found that kids who grow up in homes with dogs have lower rates of asthma, allergies, and eczema than kids without dogs. One reason for this may be that dogs actually bring microbial diversity to a family. When scientists analyze the microbes in the guts of dog owners, they find that humans pick up some of their dogs' gut microbes. And families tend to share more microbes among each other when they have a dog—probably because dogs transport microbes from family member to family member through licking and cuddling.

We know that having a dog is associated with a lower risk of heart disease. This may be because dog owners tend to walk more, and because companionship with an animal reduces human stress levels. But who knows—maybe your pup's Little Buddies are helping your ticker, too.

What it all comes down to is this: Most of us can let up a bit on the cleaning and disinfecting. Although there definitely are times to be careful about germs, we don't have to make dirt our number one public enemy. Who would have ever thought that getting dirty would be a doctor-recommended prescription for good health?

Coming Up

Now that we've taken a good look at all of the ways you can protect, support, and increase your beneficial microbes, it's time to get down to details. Next up: *The Lose Your Belly Diet* and meal plans.

PART
IV

The Lose Your Belly Diet Plan, Meal Plans, and Weight Loss Maintenance Guide

We've covered a lot of ground so far. Now we're going to get down to brass tacks and talk about the specific daily eating plans that will help protect and support your gut microbes while helping you lose weight, reduce your risk of disease, and feel more energetic every day.

This plan makes it wonderfully easy to pump up the fibre in your diet to feed the beneficial bacteria in your gut. In fact, it contains *unlimited* amounts of the superstar foods that nourish gut bacteria. It contains various kinds of fibre from different kinds of plant foods, including vegetables, fruits, pulses, nuts, and seeds. Not only does fibre feed your Little Buddies, but it fills you up while helping you slim down and maintain weight loss. With all the fibre that this plan contains, it's nearly impossible to feel hungry.

You'll also be eating the fantastic probiotic foods I've been talking about in this book. If you haven't tried all of these probiotic foods, don't worry—until recently, I hadn't tried them all, either. I've always been a huge fan of yogurt, but some of the other probiotic foods were new to me. I gave them a try and now I love them—and I think you will, too.

The Lose Your Belly Diet is easy to follow because it comes down to just five simple guidelines:

1. **Enjoy probiotic foods every day.** Probiotic foods deliver living bacteria to your gut. The most well-known of these is yogurt, but

there are others I wrote about earlier, such as kefir, kimchi, and live-culture sauerkraut, and they're an important part of *The Lose Your Belly Diet*. Each day, I recommend eating one or more live-culture or fermented foods.

2. **Eat an abundance of Prebiotic Superstars.** Prebiotics are different from probiotics in that they don't contain live and active cultures, but they do promote the health of gut bacteria by feeding them the nutrient they need most: dietary fibre. Certain prebiotic foods in the diet—I refer to them as Prebiotic Superstars—are so beneficial to gut bacteria that they can be eaten at *any time*. There's no need to consciously limit these super healthy foods.

3. **Pick a mix of proteins.** High-protein foods help chase away hunger and bring about successful weight loss, so you'll eat a healthy amount of them as part of this plan. But I don't just want you eating your usual go-to meat and poultry proteins. Your Little Buddies love plant proteins! My pick-your-protein plan makes it easy to include a wide variety of all kinds of protein foods in your meals and snacks.

4. **Choose great grains.** Grains are back! If you've been cutting out breads and other grains because you heard they weren't good for you, I'm happy to tell you that you don't have to do that anymore. Science has sided with whole grains, not just for gut health but for weight loss as well. My programme includes a great mix of grains that you can enjoy every day.

5. **Embrace friendly fats.** Like grains, fats have been pushed for years to the side of the table, but I'm happy to tell you that you can start eating fat again. Healthy fats play a very important (and tasty) role in this plan.

There you have it—that's *The Lose Your Belly Diet* in a nutshell. Now that I've given you an overview, we'll drill down a bit and look at details about food choices and portion sizes for each of my Five Gut Guidelines. But first—I'd like you to spend just a few minutes documenting how you feel before you start your new plan for healthy eating by taking two simple quizzes.

The Lose Your Belly Diet Quizzes

Following *The Lose Your Belly Diet* will definitely help support and protect your gut bacteria. And it may help you lose weight. But here's some more great news: it may also help you feel better throughout the day.

Many people find that this plan helps reduce their minor GI symptoms—no surprise there, since it provides an abundance of nutritious foods that are just what your gut needs to feel great. But this plan goes beyond gut health. Often, people who follow *The Lose Your Belly Diet* also find that they sleep better, are more energetic, and feel calmer and less stressed.

I'm sure you're revving to get started, but before you dive in, I've put together two very brief quizzes that will help you know exactly where your baseline is before you start. Then, I'm going to ask you to repeat these quizzes each week for six weeks. Doing so will help you chart your progress and see how much better you're feeling as you move forward. I don't just want you to lose excess pounds; I want you to feel better in every way!

Quiz 1: Big Picture Health Check

Directions: *For each question, choose the number that best fits how you have felt overall during the past week. Each question uses a 10-point scale.*

SLEEP: On a scale of 0–10, where 0 is "terrible sleep" and 10 is "amazing sleep," circle the number that shows how well you slept most of the week.

Terrible sleep									Amazing sleep	
0	1	2	3	4	5	6	7	8	9	10

ENERGY: Circle the number that shows how energetic you felt this week.

No energy									Abundant energy	
0	1	2	3	4	5	6	7	8	9	10

MOOD: Circle the number that shows how your mood has been this week.

Cranky, anxious, and blue									Walking on sunshine	
0	1	2	3	4	5	6	7	8	9	10

MENTAL CLARITY/BRAIN FOG: Circle the number that shows how clear your thinking and memory have been this week.

Foggy and jumbled									Crystal clear and focused	
0	1	2	3	4	5	6	7	8	9	10

STRESS: Circle the number that shows how you coped with stress.

Stress mess									Cool, calm, and totally chilled	
0	1	2	3	4	5	6	7	8	9	10

Scoring: Add up the numbers you circled. (Your score will be between 0 and 50.) This is your **Big Picture Health Score.** Write your score in the following chart, which you'll use to keep track of how you feel over time. Repeat at the end of each week.

Weekly Big Picture Health Chart

Timing	Date	Your Big Picture Health Score (0–50)	Notes In this space, write down anything that may have affected your score for that week, such as an illness, a business trip that interfered with your eating plan, etc.
Pre-Diet			
Week 1			
Week 2			
Week 3			
Week 4			
Week 5			
Week 6			

Quiz 2: GI Health Check

Directions: *For each question, choose the number that best fits how you have felt overall during the past week. Each question uses a 10-point scale.*

INDIGESTION: Circle the number that shows how often you experienced indigestion.

Lots of indigestion								No indigestion at all		
0	1	2	3	4	5	6	7	8	9	10

BLOATING AND WIND: Circle the number that shows how often you've experienced abdominal bloating and wind.

Balloon belly								No bloating at all		
0	1	2	3	4	5	6	7	8	9	10

CRAMPING: Circle the number that shows how often you've experienced abdominal cramping.

Ouch, ouch, ouch!								No cramping at all		
0	1	2	3	4	5	6	7	8	9	10

NAUSEA: Circle the number that shows how often you've experienced nausea.

Get me to the bathroom								No nausea at all		
0	1	2	3	4	5	6	7	8	9	10

QUALITY OF BOWEL MOVEMENTS: Circle the number that shows how your bowel movements have been.

Significant constipation or diarrhoea								Smooth moves		
0	1	2	3	4	5	6	7	8	9	10

Scoring: Add up the numbers you circled. (Your score will be between 0 and 50.) This is your **GI Health Score.** Write your score in the following chart, which you'll use to keep track of how you feel over time. Repeat at the end of each week.

Weekly GI Health Chart

Timing	Date	Your GI Health Score (0–50)	Notes In this space, write down anything that may have affected your score for that week, such as an illness, a business trip that interfered with your eating plan, etc.
Pre-Diet			
Week 1			
Week 2			
Week 3			
Week 4			
Week 5			
Week 6			

If your GI Health Score is not improving, I would recommend discussing this with your healthcare provider, as you could have a specific food sensitivity, intolerance, or some other health issues that may require an individualized approach.

Make sure you fill in these two charts every week so that you can keep an eye on your great progress!

The Lose Your Belly Diet Guidelines

Now that you've charted your Big Picture health and your GI health, let's look more closely at *The Lose Your Belly Diet*'s Five Gut Guidelines.

Gut Guideline #1

Enjoy Probiotic Foods Every Day

Servings per day: 1 or more

As we discussed back in chapter 10, probiotic foods are foods that actually deliver living bacteria into your body. When you eat probiotic foods, which are teeming with helpful bacteria, you add to the number and diversity of bacteria in your gut. I recommend that you include at least one probiotic food in your daily menu each day.

Yogurt is the most well-known probiotic food, but there are others as well, such as kefir, kimchi, kombucha, miso, and tempeh.

Try to go for variety when it comes to eating the recommended probiotic foods, since different kinds deliver different kinds of microbes. So, for example, have yogurt one day, kefir the next, kimchi the next—you get the idea. Or if you enjoy having yogurt for breakfast most days of the week, have other probiotic foods at other times of the day. You can also eat different brands of probiotic foods, because they may contain different strains of bacteria.

Probiotic dairy foods: Yogurt (regular, drinkable, or Greek), kefir.

- ▸ Serving size: 230g of regular yogurt, drinkable yogurt, or kefir, or 140–170g of Greek yogurt.

- Dairy probiotics also count as a protein serving.

- Choose full-fat yogurt (preferably organic, made from milk from grass-fed cows) or low-fat if you prefer the taste.

Probiotic vegetables: Kimchi, sauerkraut.

- Serving size: ½ cup

Probiotic soya foods: Tempeh, miso.

- Serving size: 85g

- Soya foods also count as a protein serving

Gut Guideline #2

Eat an Abundance of Prebiotic Superstars

Servings per day: Unlimited

Some foods are so beneficial for gut bacteria (and the rest of your body, too) that you can eat them any time. These foods are referred to as Prebiotic Superstars (pre = "before" and biotic = "life") because they are fantastic sources of the soluble and insoluble fibre that support the life of your Little Buddies. Include these high-fibre Prebiotic Superstars in meals and snacks, and nibble on them whenever you're hungry to feed yourself and your gut.

Prebiotic Superstar Veggies: *All* vegetables, from A–Z, and everything in between.

- Serving size: 1 cup of raw leafy greens, ½ cup of other raw vegetables, or ½ cup cooked vegetables.

- Aim to have a *minimum* of 6–7 servings of Superstar Veggies per day. But have as many as you want, because there's no limit!

- Eat a wide variety of different types and colours of vegetables.

- Cooked veggies are fine sometimes, but your gut bacteria live best on raw veggies, so eat them whenever you can. (If, like me, you're not crazy about plain raw veggies, I'll help you dress them up and make them more enjoyable. Your mouth will water for my flavourful chow-chow recipes and all the delicious dips and healthy dressings in the recipe section.)

▸ The only limit is on starchy vegetables (corn, green lima beans, peas, sweet potatoes, potatoes, taro, and water chestnuts), which are best kept to ½ cup total per day.

Prebiotic Superstar Fruits: All fruits contain fibre and nutrients. But a few are true superstars because they're flush with fibre and relatively low in sugar. Apples, pears, blueberries, blackberries, raspberries, and mixed berries (a mix of blueberries, blackberries, raspberries, and strawberries) are so good for your gut bacteria that I want you to make them a big part of your diet.

▸ Serving size: 1 cup of berries or 1 medium-size apple or pear.

▸ Aim to have a minimum of 2 servings of Superstar Fruits per day. But don't feel you have to limit yourself to 2 servings. Obviously you want to be sensible and not eat the entire fruit stand, but high-fibre fruit is not why we are facing an obesity epidemic in this country. Enjoy several servings a day!

▸ You'll notice that strawberries are not considered Superstar Fruits, but mixed berries—which include strawberries—are. I'm not losing my marbles—there really is a good reason for this. When it comes to berries, strawberries have less fibre and more sugar than other kinds, so I don't think it's a good idea to eat them in unlimited amounts. But they're fine when combined with other higher-fibre berries, as they are in the bags of frozen mixed berries I like to buy for smoothies.

▸ As for other fruits: It's not going to kill you to eat fruits that aren't on this Superstar list. But I leave them off the list because most are lower in fibre and higher in sugar than Superstar Fruits, and these are important considerations when you're trying to feed your gut and lose weight. If you'd like to have a banana, peach, orange, plum, some melon, or other fruit, it's fine. But I like to keep things simple, and the simplest, most effective initial approach for weight loss and gut health is to focus on the Superstar Fruits. You should add in other fruits after you reach your weight-loss goals and are maintaining your healthy weight.

Drink Up

Fluids are an important part of *The Lose Your Belly Diet*. As you add more fibre to your daily eating plan, you need enough fluid to keep that fibre moving through your system so you don't get constipated. Have a 230ml cup of water, coffee, or tea with each meal or snack and aim for a total of at least 8 cups a day (there is no hard science to back this amount up, but it's a nice baseline to shoot for). Don't worry about coffee bothering your Little Buddies—studies suggest that moderate amounts of coffee are actually beneficial to gut bacteria. Just avoid the added sugars and don't overdo it on the caffeine. If you want anything in your coffee, I'd much rather you go with a splash of semi-skimmed milk rather than a bunch of sweetener.

Gut Guideline #3

Pick a Mix of Proteins

Servings per day: 6–7

Your gut bacteria thrive on high-fibre foods, but your body also needs ample amounts of protein for good health and weight loss. I know people have different preferences when it comes to protein: some like meat; others prefer plant proteins. As I've noted, I take a flexitarian approach that includes primarily plant and occasionally meat sources.

Although it's fine to include some beef, pork, poultry, and lamb in your diet, you're better off relying mostly on fish, dairy, nuts, and pulses to meet your protein needs. I recommend eating plant-based protein sources several times a day. These include nuts, seeds, pulses, and soya foods.

If you're a meat lover, a great way to do this is to have smaller amounts of meat along with foods that contain plant proteins—think beefy chilli with beans, for example, or veggie-grain dishes in which meat is more of a side than the centre of the meal. Mix things up and choose a total of 6–7 servings of all kinds of protein each day, with most of it coming from nonmeat sources. I ideally recommend including one source of protein in every meal and snack.

And please keep this in mind as you buy any animal products, including meat, fish, poultry, eggs, and milk. As we discussed in chapter 11, it is best for your Little Buddies to eat foods that are raised in ways that support our health, so whenever possible, choose animal products that are grass-fed, organic, and raised without antibiotics.

Nut/seed protein: Nuts and seeds provide the protein you need and the fibre your Little Buddies love. Enjoy almonds, walnuts, peanuts, pecans, pistachios, and other nuts, as well as pumpkin, sesame, sunflower, and other seeds.

- ▶ Serving size: 1 tablespoon nut butter, 2 tablespoons (30g) nuts, 2 tablespoons (30g) seeds.

Pulses protein: Beans, peas, and lentils deliver loads of fibre as well as protein. And they're way cheaper (and better for the planet) than meat.

- ▶ Serving size: ½ cup cooked pulses, or 3 tablespoons hummus.

Dairy protein: In addition to protein, dairy foods provide calcium, vitamin D, and other nutrients.

- ▶ Serving size: 1 cup of milk, regular yogurt, drinkable yogurt, or kefir, 140–170g Greek yogurt, 30g hard cheese, ½ cup soft cheese such as ricotta or cottage cheese, or 2 small wedges of spreadable cheese such as Laughing Cow. Choose dairy made from cow's milk or goat's milk.
- ▶ Whenever possible, choose dairy foods from sources that are grass-fed, organic, and raised without antibiotics.
- ▶ Keep in mind that almond milk isn't a good substitute for dairy milk, because when it comes to protein, it doesn't contain much. It's fine to have it, but don't rely on it as a protein source. If you do buy it, choose unflavoured, unsweetened varieties.

Egg protein: Eggs are an excellent source of protein as well as several vitamins.

- ▶ Serving size: 2 medium eggs.
- ▶ You'll notice I suggest whole eggs and not egg whites. This is based on new information about eggs. Particularly when it comes to organic eggs, we are starting to realize the yolk may actually be good for you. If you still want to cut back on egg yolks, you can substitute

3 egg whites for 1 whole egg. However, I don't recommend this for most folks because egg yolks are a nice source of vitamin A and some helpful antioxidants, and most of the research linking egg yolks to heart disease has not held up. In my case, as I've switched from egg whites to whole eggs and increased my healthy fat intake in general, my cholesterol profile has actually improved.

► Buy healthier eggs—look for organic eggs that are raised without hormones or added antibiotics, from hens fed vegetarian diets rich in omega-3 fatty acids. These eggs are better for you and your gut than factory-raised conventional eggs. And they tend to taste better, too!

Veggie burger protein: I am a huge fan of veggie burgers for a quick meal. Not only do they contain protein, but their veggie ingredients add fibre and nutrients such as vitamins A and C. These are an excellent, tasty substitute for meat. Be sure to choose veggie burgers whose first few ingredients are vegetables, not soya protein.

► Serving size: 1 veggie burger.

Soya protein: Tofu and tempeh are good substitutes for meat, and tempeh has the added bonus of being a probiotic food.

► Serving size: 85g tempeh or tofu.

Seafood protein: Fish and shellfish contain protein as well as omega-3 fatty acids and other nutrients.

► Serving sizes: 55–85g fatty fish (anchovies, herring, mackerel, salmon, sardines, swordfish, trout, tuna), 115g lean white fish (cod, sole, flounder, haddock, canned tuna in water, sea bass), or 115g shellfish (prawns, crab, lobster, oysters, scallops).

► Note that serving sizes of higher-fat, higher-calorie fish are smaller than that of lower-fat, lower-calorie fish.

Poultry protein: Chicken and turkey are a source of protein and some other important nutrients.

► Serving size: 85–115g.

Protein Powders

If you're in the habit of adding protein powder to smoothies, you may be wondering whether you should continue doing this while following *The Lose Your Belly Diet*. I believe that protein powders are not really necessary when you are eating a balanced diet. Unless you are a bodybuilder, you get all the protein you need from a healthy diet that includes protein foods in each meal and snack.

If you do decide to add protein powder to smoothies, choose unflavoured powders that are either whey- or plant-based (pea protein or a plant protein blend). Count a scoop of protein powder (100–120 calories) as 1 serving of protein.

Meat protein: Beef, pork, lamb, and venison provide some nutrients that aren't found in plant proteins, such as vitamin B12, and are good sources of iron.

- Serving size: 55–85g.
- Note that serving sizes of meat are smaller than that of lower-calorie proteins.
- Avoid processed meat that is smoked, salted, or cured.
- Grilling can add cancer-causing compounds to meat; opt for baking, sautéing, poaching, stir-frying, and braising as much as possible.
- Whenever possible, choose meats that are grass-fed, organic, and raised without antibiotics.

Protein bars: I know a lot of people who rely on protein bars for on-the-go snacks and meals. I know I do—I travel a lot, so I've always got them in my bag. It's best to eat healthy, whole foods. But when you're strapped for time, the right kind of protein bar can make a good snack or meal replacement. I like lower-sugar nut bars, because, for the most part, they have healthy ingredients and not too much added sugar.

- Serving size: 1 bar.

- In general, choose nut-based bars which are high in protein (at least 5 grams), low in sugar (ideally 5 grams or less), and contain around 200 calories or less.

- If you're allergic to nuts, oat-based protein bars are an option, although many are lower in protein and higher in sugar. Check the label to see if the bar was made in a facility that also processes nuts.

- Watch out for protein bars made with dried fruit, because they tend to be high in sugar.

- To turn a protein bar into a meal, pair it with fruit or a salad.

- Most protein bars will count as 1 protein and 1 fat. (More on fats below.)

Gut Guideline #4

Choose Great Grains

Servings per day: 2–3

Whole grains are another excellent source of dietary fibre. We've heard a lot of grumbling about carbohydrates in past years, but further study has shown that the problem is with processed "white" foods made with grains that have been stripped of their fibre and nutrients. There's no reason to hide from whole grains—in fact, they are an excellent food for your gut bacteria. Just be sure to choose whole grains, such as whole-wheat bread or quinoa, rather than processed grains, such as white bread or white rice. When buying breads, pasta, or snack foods, be sure the first ingredient on the label is a whole grain. And don't bother with it if it is high in sugar.

Serving sizes:

- 1 slice whole-grain bread

- 1 whole-grain English muffin

- ½ cup cooked, unsweetened oatmeal

Dr. T's Tasty Tip

Believe it or not, I'm okay with you eating crisps—as long as they're the right kind of crisps. We really are in a new era of healthy crisps. As a result you can now enjoy a wide variety of crisps that are much healthier than you could have ever imagined even 10 years ago.

My personal favourite are made from beans, which means they are plentiful in fibre, protein, and other nutrients. And all of their ingredients are things that you will recognize. They can be a challenge to find so when I discover them in a shop, I stock up on a few bags.

When you choose healthy crisps, make sure the ingredients are real foods. Look for crisps whose first ingredient is a whole grain or beans.

- ¾ cup whole-grain cold cereal
- ¼ cup granola
- ½ cup cooked whole grains such as amaranth, barley, brown rice, buckwheat, bulgur, farro, millet, or quinoa
- 30g whole-grain crackers
- 3 cups of plain, air-popped popcorn
- ½ cup cooked whole-wheat pasta (30g uncooked)
- 1 small whole-grain tortilla
- 1 small whole-grain roll
- 100-calorie serving of whole-grain crisps

Dr. T's Shopping Tip

When buying guacamole or hummus, check out the ingredient list. If all of the ingredients are real food, you should be good to go! You can buy many different varieties today, and when possible I always opt for locally made guacamole and hummus, because they're freshest. You can also choose reduced-fat hummus.

Gut Guideline #5

Embrace Friendly Fats

Servings per day: 2–3

Healthy fats provide omega-3 fatty acids and help ward off hunger. They also help you boost your intake of vegetables, because they are a delicious ingredient in veggie dips, salad dressings, and spreads that turn raw veggies from an obligation to a treat.

Serving sizes:

- ▶ 1 tablespoon healthy oil (olive, nut, rapeseed, sesame, soybean, flaxseed, grape seed, coconut)
- ▶ 20 small or 10 large pitted black olives or green olives
- ▶ 1½–2 tablespoons oil and vinegar dressing
- ▶ ½ small or ⅓ medium avocado
- ▶ ¼ cup guacamole (with avocado as the primary ingredient)
- ▶ 1 tablespoon tahini
- ▶ 100-calorie square of dark chocolate (chocolate with 70 percent or more cacao)
- ▶ Some diet plans count nuts and seeds as fats *or* proteins, but this plan doesn't do that. I think it makes more sense to count nuts and seeds only as proteins, because this makes it easier for you to eat more plant-based protein and less animal protein. Also, it frees up your fat servings for salad dressings, veggie dips, and other "veggie helpers" that make it easier for you to eat more raw veggies, which your gut bacteria love.

A Range of Choices

You'll notice that for some of the five guidelines, I give a range of daily servings. That's because people's bodies are different and our weight management goals are different. There's no such thing as a one-size-fits-all eating plan. A sedentary woman who is 5 feet 2 inches needs less food than an active man who happens to be 6 feet 4. Also, someone who's trying to lose a significant amount of weight would want to eat less than someone who doesn't have as much weight to lose. And if you're very active, you need ample fuel to keep your body going.

I'm all about keeping things simple, so I'm giving you two versions of *The Lose Your Belly Diet*: Lose Your Belly EXPRESS and Lose Your Belly EXTRA. Both plans include the same super-healthy foods, but the serving amounts are adjusted to reflect your body size, goals, activity levels, and other factors.

Lose Your Belly EXPRESS: You may want to follow the EXPRESS Plan if you feel that you'd meet your goals more effectively by eating a smaller amount of food. For example, EXPRESS might be for you if you have more than 20 pounds to lose, if you have a smaller frame, if you are fairly sedentary, or if you have a slower metabolism because of age, health, or menopausal status.

Lose Your Belly EXTRA: You may want to follow the EXTRA Plan if you need a little more food than is offered in the EXPRESS Plan—for example, if you have a larger frame, if you are fairly active, if you have fewer than 20 pounds to lose, or you know you have a fast metabolism. You can even switch back and forth between EXPRESS and EXTRA on a day-by-day basis. Some people cycle from one to the other on alternate days. Or they follow the EXTRA Plan when they do a lot of activity and EXPRESS when they have a less-active day. Or they stick with EXPRESS most of the time, but turn to EXTRA when they're having an extra-hungry day or a high-stress day. This is a great idea, because it helps you feed that extra hunger with gut-healthy foods rather than the sugary snack foods you may have grabbed in the past when your stomach growled. Follow whichever plan seems right for you—you know your body best, and you know what your weight-loss goals are.

For quicker results: If you want to accelerate weight loss even more, you have the option of limiting fruit to 1–2 servings a day and cutting back on whole grains for the first few weeks that you're following the plan. Although these are healthy foods that are important for your health and the health of your Little Buddies, cutting back slightly in the beginning can help kick-start weight loss in a way that can be very motivating for some people. But don't starve yourself, and don't eliminate whole groups of food. I know it's satisfying to get results quickly, but you don't want to starve your Little Buddies of the high-fibre foods they need to live.

Here's a simple wrap-up of how many servings each of the plans includes:

Food	Lose Your Belly EXPRESS Daily serving goals	Lose Your Belly EXTRA Daily serving goals
Prebiotic Superstar Fruits and Veggies	Unlimited (at least 2 servings of Superstar Fruits and 6 servings of Superstar Veggies)	Unlimited (at least 2 servings of Superstar Fruits and 7 servings of Superstar Veggies)
Probiotic Foods	1 or more servings daily (count dairy in protein tally)	1 or more servings daily (count dairy in protein tally)
Proteins	6 servings	7 servings
Whole Grains	2 servings	3 servings
Fats	2 servings	3 servings

The Lose Your Belly Diet, Meal by Meal

The Lose Your Belly Diet is meant to be flexible, but I find that most people do best when they take a traditional three meals/two snacks approach that distributes protein and other foods fairly evenly throughout the day. One of the most important elements to any successful eating plan is to stave off hunger, and I have found that for most people, spreading food out over the course of the day helps maintain energy levels and satiety.

If you prefer to structure your daily menu in a different way, that's fine with me—you know your body way better than I do, and this diet is flexible enough that you can make it work for you no matter how you like to eat. But unless you have a strong pull in another direction, I recommend three meals and two snacks daily. In general, I recommend that you eat something—either a meal or a snack—every three or four hours or so.

As you follow the plan, keep this in mind: It's very important to pay attention to portion sizes if you're trying to lose weight or maintain weight loss. Even if you eat the healthiest diet in the world, you're not going to lose weight if you eat way too many calories every day.

To make sure you're hitting the nail on the head with portion sizes, you've got to measure your food. This isn't hard to do—invest a few bucks in a set of measuring spoons and a measuring cup, and you'll be good to go. You can also buy an inexpensive kitchen scale—it's such an easy way to keep track of what you're eating. Then, when you're preparing a meal, you can easily measure your food so you know you're getting the right amount.

Don't worry, you won't have to measure your foods forever—soon you'll learn the correct portion sizes of the foods you eat regularly and your body will tell you the right amount of food it needs to satisfy your hunger without over-eating. But to start, make sure you're getting the right portion sizes of food, because distorted eyeballing can easily interfere with weight loss.

I'm also recommending that you track what you eat. You won't have to do this forever, either—eventually you'll become so familiar with the guidelines that you'll follow them automatically. And you don't have to list all the foods you eat—although you certainly can if you want, because this does help some people with a sense of accountability. But do track the number of servings of each food you eat, at least for the first few weeks, because it really does help you build healthy new habits.

I've included an easy Food Tracker on page 154 you can use. Or feel free to do your own tracking on your phone, in a notebook, on a whiteboard hung in your kitchen, or even on a sticky note on your desk. It doesn't matter what you use—write it with lipstick on your bathroom mirror if you want—just as long as you keep track.

A Note about Alcohol

For the first four weeks that you follow *The Lose Your Belly Diet*, I recommend avoiding alcohol because doing so can help jump-start weight loss. Beginning in week 5, feel free to have 2 servings a week on the EXPRESS Plan and

5–7 servings per week on the EXTRA Plan (maximum one drink per day). A serving of alcohol is 350ml of beer, 150ml of wine, or 45ml of spirits (i.e., the amount it takes to fill a standard shot glass). If you go with spirits, a safe bet is vodka with unsweetened soda water and a wedge of lime or other fruit. The calories and sugar in mixed drinks can add up very quickly. Also, never be afraid to tell a barman exactly how you want a drink made because all too often they add in a bunch of sweeteners that can wreck your progress.

Count an alcoholic beverage as a serving of grains. I know it may seem silly but when it comes to calories I count any kind of alcohol as a grain because it is composed mainly of carbohydrates, just as grains are. Obviously, wine, beer, and alcohol are not whole grains, but it makes the most sense to track them as grains so you don't forget that alcohol indeed contains significant calories.

Your Tracking Sheet

Directions: *Use this chart to keep track of the number of servings of each kind of food you eat at meals and snacks.*

	Break-fast	Snack #1	Lunch	Snack #2	Dinner	Day's Total
Superstar Fruit Servings (daily target: at least 2 servings)						
Superstar Veggie Servings (daily target: at least 6–7 servings)						
Protein Servings (daily target: 6–7 servings)						
Grain Servings (daily target: 2–3 servings)						
Fat Servings (daily target: 2–3 servings)						
Probiotic Servings (daily target: 1 or more servings)						
Water, Coffee, or Tea (daily target: 8 cups fluid total)						

Dr. T's Shortcut to a Healthy Day

On some days I don't have the time to focus on food prep or even sitting down for formal meals. Whether you are solo or cooking for a family, you know how easy it is to fall off the healthy meal train on certain days.

But there is absolutely no need to stress. I have discovered easy shortcuts that keep me healthy even when I don't have the time or energy for full-on meals. The key: quick, easy meals that can feed one person or the whole crew.

There are plenty of recipes in this book that fit the bill but below are examples of the types of foods I eat on a busy day. Truth be told, it feels like a cheat day, but I still eat healthily and feel good at the end of the day. My motto: we can't always control our schedule, but we can always control what we put in our bodies.

▸ Breakfast on the go: Low-sugar nut bar (5g sugar)

▸ Mid-morning snack: Apple with nut butter (almond or cashew), or yogurt with raspberries or blueberries

▸ Microwave lunch: Spicy veggie burger on whole-grain bread with hummus, avocado or guacamole, and/or mustard. Or, I have an low-sodium veggie burger topped with sauerkraut and mustard on a bed of fresh spinach plus/minus organic cheese.

▸ Afternoon snack: Handful of mixed nuts or cashews (my personal favourite) with 30g grass-fed cheddar cheese

▸ Pre-dinner: A glass of red wine or a beer. More hops mean more calories, but it also means a higher content of polyphenols, which are powerful antioxidants. And in horses at least, researchers think hops may help control gut microbial imbalances!

▸ Dinner: Amazing 1 Minute Bean Burrito or Split Second Veggie Nachos (see page 92).

▸ Guilty yet healthy pleasure: 85 percent dark chocolate square with almond butter. This dessert has heart-healthy fats and gut-benefiting fibre. When I first started eating dark chocolate, I had some adjusting to do, and it took me some time to work up to 85 percent dark chocolate. But now it's actually what I prefer.

Meal Planning Guides

This diet has lots of flexibility, and you can build your meals however you like. Start with protein. I recommend a serving or two of protein with each meal or snack. Add in an abundance of Superstar Fruits and Veggies at every meal and snack. Use your fats where you need them—in my case, I tend to pair them up with veggies, because I enjoy raw veggies much more with some kind of a dressing or dip that contains fat. Finally, slot in your whole grains, planning them for the meals or snacks where you tend to feel most hungry.

Below are sample daily frameworks you can use for your daily meal planning. Feel free to tweak them as you see fit—other than having protein at each meal and snack, it's up to you to distribute your servings however you like. Just keep an eye on your daily targets and you'll be fine.

Lose Your Belly EXPRESS
Daily Meal Planning Guide

Lose Your Belly EXPRESS Daily Serving Total:

- ▸ Unlimited Superstar Fruits (at least 2)
- ▸ Unlimited Superstar Veggies (at least 6)
- ▸ 6 Proteins
- ▸ 2 Whole Grains
- ▸ 2 Fats

Lose Your Belly EXPRESS
Sample Daily Meal Plan

Breakfast	1 Protein + Superstar Fruits/Veggies
Lunch	1 Protein + 1 Whole Grain + Superstar Fruits/Veggies
Dinner	2 Protein + 1 Whole Grain + 1 Fat + Superstar Fruits/Veggies
Snack #1	1 Protein + Superstar Fruits/Veggies
Snack #2	1 Protein + 1 Fat + Superstar Fruits/Veggies

Lose Your Belly EXTRA
Daily Meal Planning Guide

Lose Your Belly EXTRA Daily Serving Total:

- ▸ Unlimited Superstar Fruits (at least 2)
- ▸ Unlimited Superstar Veggies (at least 7)
- ▸ 7 Proteins
- ▸ 3 Whole Grains
- ▸ 3 Fats

Lose Your Belly EXTRA
Sample Daily Meal Plan

Breakfast	1 Protein + 1 Whole Grain + Superstar Fruits/Veggies
Lunch	2 Protein + 1 Whole Grain + 1 Fat + Superstar Fruits/Veggies
Dinner	2 Protein + 1 Whole Grain + 1 Fat + Superstar Fruits/Veggies
Snack #1	1 Protein + Superstar Fruits/Veggies
Snack #2	1 Protein + 1 Fat + Superstar Fruits/Veggies

Maintaining Weight Loss

Once you meet your weight-loss goals, you can continue to follow the principles of *The Lose Your Belly Diet*, adjusting it as needed to help you stay on track. We'll talk more about that later, but in general, I'll recommend that you keep your focus on eating an abundance of superstar foods while adding in other fruits and perhaps an extra serving of protein, whole grains, or healthy fats.

Daily Meal Plan Menu

Some people like to plan their own menus; others prefer to follow the plan I've created. Either is fine, as long as you make sure you're getting the right number of servings of food each day. If you use the following menu plan, keep a few things in mind:

▶ This daily menu is for the Lose Your Belly EXPRESS Plan. If you follow Lose Your Belly EXTRA, make sure to add in the additional EXTRA servings.

▶ Menu items in bold have recipes included at the end of this book. But make sure to check out all the recipes, because only a sampling of them are featured in the following menus.

▶ This menu is designed as a traditional breakfast-lunch-dinner style, with soups and salads at lunch and main dishes at dinner. But if you'd prefer to switch it up, go right ahead. Have breakfast foods for dinner, lunch for dinner—whatever works for you.

▶ In my menus I've scheduled snacks for mid-morning and mid-afternoon. But you can go ahead and have snacks when you need them, during your hungriest time—mid-morning, mid-afternoon, or evening.

WEEK 1

	Breakfast	Snack #1	Lunch	Snack #2	Dinner
Day 1	1 c blueberries; 1 serving yogurt (1 fruit, 1 protein)	Apple spread with 1 tbs nut butter (1 fruit, 1 protein)	**Chicken and Avocado Salad** (2½ veggies, 2 proteins, 1 fat)	30g whole-grain crackers; 30g sliced cheddar cheese (1 protein, 1 grain)	**Quinoa-Stuffed Peppers**; side salad (1 c greens, ½ c other veggies) with 2 tbs **Simple Vinaigrette** (5½ veggies, 1 protein, 1 grain, 1 fat)
Day 2	¾ c whole-grain cereal with 1 c milk or kefir; 1 c raspberries (1 fruit, 1 protein, 1 grain)	Sliced pear; 2 tbs almonds (1 fruit, 1 protein)	**Spinach and Egg Salad** (3 veggies, 2 proteins, 1 fat)	1 c raw veggies dipped in ¼ c guacamole (2 veggies, 1 fat)	**Fast and Easy Turkey Chilli**; ½ c kimchi or live-culture sauerkraut; ½ c cooked brown rice (4 veggies, 2 proteins, 1 grain)
Day 3	**Berry Smoothie** (1 fruit, 1 protein)	KIND bar and an apple (1 fruit, 1 protein, 1 fat)	**Hearty Lentil Soup;** 30g whole-grain crackers (1½ veggies, 1 protein, 1 grain)	1 c raw veggies dipped in 3 tbs hummus (2 veggies, 1 protein)	**Beef Stir-Fry** (including optional grains); side salad (1 c greens, ½ c other veggies) with **Rosemary Garlic Dressing** (5 veggies, 2 proteins, 1 grain, 1 fat)
Day 4	**Pizza Omelette**; 1 c mixed berries (1 fruit, 2 veggies, 2 proteins)	1 serving yogurt mixed with 1 apple, chopped, and cinnamon (1 fruit, 1 protein)	**Easy Chicken Barley Soup** (1½ veggies, 1 protein, 1 grain)	**Mediterranean Chow-Chow;** 1 square dark chocolate (2 veggies, 1 fat)	**Loaded Veggie Burger**; ½ c kimchi or live-culture sauerkraut; side salad (1 c greens, ½ c other veggies) with **Lemony Dill Dressing** (4 veggies, 2 proteins, 1 grain, 1 fat)
Day 5	**Granola Yogurt** (1 fruit, 1 protein, 1 grain)	KIND bar and an apple (1 fruit, 1 protein, 1 fat)	**Farmer's Market Chopped Salad** (6 veggies, 1 protein, 1 fat)	1 c cherry tomatoes dipped in ½ c ricotta cheese mixed with chopped fresh basil (2 veggies, 1 protein)	115g baked chicken; **Salsa Beans;** ½ c cooked quinoa (½ veggie, 2 proteins, 1 grain)
Day 6	½ c oatmeal made with water; ½ c cottage cheese topped with 1 pear, chopped (1 fruit, 1 protein, 1 grain)	**Fruity Veggie Smoothie** (1 fruit, ½ veggie, 1 protein)	**Loaded Veggie Burger** (1 veggie, 2 proteins, 1 grain, 1 fat)	30g cheddar cheese; **Summer Harvest Chow-Chow** (1 protein, 2 veggies)	115g baked haddock; side salad (1 c greens, ½ c other veggies) with **Rosemary Garlic Dressing** (2 veggies, 1 protein, 1 fat)
Day 7	Whole-grain toast with 1 tbs nut butter; 1 apple (1 fruit, 1 protein, 1 grain)	**Nutty Berry Smoothie** (1 fruit, 2 protein)	115g tuna; side salad (1 c greens, ½ c other veggies) with **Lemony Dill Dressing** (2 veggies, 1 protein)	1 c raw veggies dipped in ½ c salsa; 1 square dark chocolate (3 veggies, 1 fat)	**Bulgur with Spinach, Tomatoes, White Beans, and Feta Cheese** (1½ veggies, 2 proteins, 1 grain, 1 fat)

WEEK 2

	Breakfast	Snack #1	Lunch	Snack #2	Dinner
Day 1	2 scrambled eggs; 1 slice whole-grain toast; 1 sliced pear (1 fruit, 1 protein, 1 grain)	**Berry Smoothie** (1 fruit, 1 protein)	115g prawns with a side salad (1 c greens, ½ c other veggies) with **Rosemary Garlic Dressing** (2 veggies, 1 protein)	1 tbs nuts; 1 c sliced cucumbers dipped in **Green Goddess Dip** (2 veggies, 1 fat, 1 protein)	**Enchiladas**; 2 c fresh spinach, steamed; (2½ veggies, 2 proteins, 1 grain, 1 fat)
Day 2	1 pear spread with 1 tbs nut butter; ½ c oatmeal made with water (1 fruit, 1 protein, 1 grain)	1 c blueberries; 1 serving yogurt (1 fruit, 1 protein)	**Tuna Salad with Chickpeas, Green Beans, and Tomatoes** (4 veggies, 2 proteins)	1 c raw veggies dipped in ¼ c guacamole (2 veggies, 1 fat)	**Loaded Veggie Burger**; side salad (1 c greens, ½ c other veggies) with **Rosemary Garlic Dressing** (3 veggies, 2 proteins, 1 grain, 1 fat)
Day 3	**Baby Greens Omelette**; 1 pear (1 fruit, 1½ veggies, 1 protein)	KIND bar and an apple (1 fruit, 1 protein, 1 fat)	**Easy Chicken Barley Soup**; ½ c kimchi or live-culture sauerkraut (2½ veggies, 1 protein, 1 grain)	1 tbs nuts; 1 c cherry tomatoes dipped in **Cool Cucumber Yogurt Dip** (2 veggies, 1 protein)	115g roast chicken; **Lentils with Barley and Spicy Tomato Sauce**; 1 square dark chocolate, (2 veggies, 2 proteins, 1 grain, 1 fat)
Day 4	1 c blackberries; 1 serving yogurt (1 fruit, 1 protein)	2 hard-boiled eggs; 1 apple, sliced, sprinkled with cinnamon (1 fruit, 1 protein)	**Cheese and Nut Salad**; 30g whole-grain crackers (5 veggies, 2 proteins, 1 grain)	½ c cottage cheese; 1 c raw veggies dipped in ¼ c guacamole (2 veggies, 1 protein, 1 fat)	**Salsa Chicken**; ½ c cooked quinoa; 1 c chopped broccoli and 1 c chopped red peppers sautéed in 1 tbs olive oil (4½ veggies, 1 protein, 1 grain, 1 fat)
Day 5	1 c blueberries; 1 serving yogurt (1 fruit, 1 protein)	2 hard-boiled eggs; 1 apple, sliced, sprinkled with cinnamon (1 fruit, 1 protein)	115g sliced chicken; side salad (1 c greens, ½ c other veggies) with **Lemony Dill Dressing** sprinkled with 2 tbs chopped walnuts; 1 square dark chocolate (2 veggies, 2 proteins, 1 fat)	30g cheddar or Gouda cheese; **South of the Border Chow-Chow** (1 protein, 2 veggies)	**Quick-Fix Spinach Lasagne**; side salad (1 c greens, ½ c other veggies) with **Tahini Dressing** (5 veggies, 1 protein, 2 grains, 1 fat)
Day 6	**Broccoli Cheddar Breakfast Burrito**; 1 c blueberries (1 fruit, 2½ veggies, 2 protein, 1 grain)	Apple, spread with 1 tbs nut butter (1 fruit, 1 protein)	**Easy Chicken Barley Soup**; ½ c chopped cucumber and ½ c chopped tomatoes tossed with **Simple Vinaigrette** (2½ veggies, 1 protein, 1 grain, 1 fat)	1 c raw veggies dipped in ½ c salsa; 1 square dark chocolate (3 veggies, 1 fat)	115–170g beef or venison; ½ c kimchi or live-culture sauerkraut; side salad (1 c greens, ½ c other veggies) with **Rosemary Garlic Dressing** (3 veggies, 2 proteins)
Day 7	**Open Breakfast Sandwich**; 1 c mixed berries (1 fruit, ½ veggie, 1 protein, 1 grain)	1 apple; 1 serving yogurt (1 fruit, 1 protein)	**Spinach and Egg Salad** (3 veggies, 2 proteins, 1 fat)	1 c cherry tomatoes dipped in **Mediterranean Ricotta Dip** (2 veggies, 1 protein, 1 fat)	115g baked cod; ½ c cooked quinoa; side salad (1 c greens, ½ c other veggies) with **Lemony Dill Dressing** (2 veggies, 1 protein, 1 grain)

WEEK 3

	Breakfast	Snack #1	Lunch	Snack #2	Dinner
Day 1	**Apple Walnut Breakfast Bowl** (1 fruit, 2 proteins)	**Berry Smoothie** (1 fruit, 1 protein)	115g tuna; side salad (1 c greens, ½ c other veggies) with **Lime Mint Dressing** (2 veggies, 1 protein)	1 c raw veggies and 30g whole-grain crackers dipped in **Homemade Hummus** (2 veggies, 1 protein, 1 grain, 1½ fat)	**Broccoli Asparagus Quinoa Salad** (3 veggies, 1 protein, 1 grain, ½ fat)
Day 2	2 scrambled eggs; 1 slice whole-grain toast; 1 sliced pear (1 fruit, 1 protein, 1 grain)	Apple, spread with 1 tbs nut butter (1 fruit, 1 protein)	**Tomato Ricotta Salad**; ½ c kimchi or live-culture sauerkraut (5½ veggies, 1 protein, 1 fat)	30g cheddar cheese; 1 c raw veggies dipped in **Coriander Lime Dressing** (2 veggies, 1 protein)	115g roast chicken; ½ c cooked black beans; **Bulgur Tabbouleh** (1 veggie, 2 proteins, 1 grain, 1 fat)
Day 3	**Cheesy Mushroom Omelette** (1½ veggies, 2 proteins)	1 c blueberries; 1 serving yogurt (1 fruit, 1 protein)	**Cinnamon Apple Salad with Pecans** (1 fruit, 2 veggies, 1 protein, 1 fat)	30g whole-grain crackers, ½ c raw carrots dipped in **Rosemary Garlic Dressing** (1 veggie, 1 grain)	115–170g beef or venison; **Roasted Root Vegetables**; 1 small whole-grain dinner roll (3 veggies, 2 proteins, 1 grain, 1 fat)
Day 4	1 pear spread with 1 tbs nut butter; ½ c oatmeal made with water (1 fruit, 1 protein, 1 grain)	KIND bar and an apple (1 fruit, 1 protein, 1 fat)	**Cheese and Nut Salad** (5 veggies, 2 proteins)	1 c raw veggies dipped in **Creamy Avocado Dressing** (2 veggies, ½ fat)	**Quinoa Veggie Pilaf**; ½ c kimchi or live-culture sauerkraut (3 veggies, 2 protein, 1 grain, ½ fat)
Day 5	**Granola Yogurt** (1 fruit, 1 protein, 1 grain)	2 hard-boiled eggs; 1 apple, sliced, sprinkled with cinnamon (1 fruit, 1 protein)	115g turkey with a side salad (1 c greens, ½ c other veggies) with **Rosemary Garlic Dressing** (2 veggies, 1 protein)	2 tbs nuts; 1 c raw veggies dipped in **Homemade Hummus** (2 veggies, 2 proteins, 1½ fat)	**Pearl Barley with Fresh Summer Veggie Sauce** (3½ veggies, 1 protein, 1 grain, ½ fat)
Day 6	1 apple spread with 1 tbs nut butter; ½ c oatmeal made with water (1 fruit, 1 protein, 1 grain)	1 c mixed berries; 1 serving yogurt (1 fruit, 1 protein)	**Green Bean Salad** (3 veggies, 2 proteins, 1 fat)	**Spring Greens Chow-Chow**; 1 square dark chocolate (2 veggies, 1 fat)	115g roasted turkey; ½ c cooked quinoa; **Salsa Beans** (½ veggie, 2 proteins, 1 grain)
Day 7	¾ c whole-grain cereal with 1 c milk or kefir; 1 c raspberries (1 fruit, 1 protein, 1 grain)	2 hard-boiled eggs; 1 apple, sliced, sprinkled with cinnamon (1 fruit, 1 protein)	Open chicken sandwich: 115g roast chicken over 1 slice whole-grain toast, topped with **Corn and Tomato Salsa** and ¼ c guacamole (1½ veggies, 1 protein, 1 grain, 1 fat)	30g cheddar cheese; 1 cherry tomatoes dipped in **Rosemary Garlic Dressing** (2 veggies, 1 protein)	**Beefy-Bean Chilli**; side salad (1 c greens, ½ c other veggies) with **Simple Vinaigrette** (4½ veggies, 2 proteins, 1 fat)

WEEK 4

	Breakfast	Snack #1	Lunch	Snack #2	Dinner
Day 1	1 c blueberries; 1 serving yogurt (1 fruit, 1 protein)	KIND bar and an apple (1 fruit, 1 protein, 1 fat)	**Easy Chicken Barley Soup** (1½ veggies, 1 protein, 1 grain)	30g cheddar cheese; 30g whole-grain crackers (1 protein, 1 grain)	**White Bean Chicken Chilli;** side salad (1 c greens, ½ c other veggies) with **Lemony Dill Dressing** (4½ veggies, 2 proteins, 1 fat)
Day 2	**Spicy Veggie Scramble** (2 veggies, 1 protein)	1 serving yogurt mixed with 1 apple, chopped, and cinnamon (1 fruit, 1 protein)	**Minestrone Soup**; 30g whole-grain crackers dipped in ¼ c guacamole (3 veggies, 1 protein, 1 grain, 1 fat)	1 c cucumber slices dipped in ½c ricotta cheese mixed with chopped fresh dill (2 veggies, 1 protein)	**Loaded Veggie Burger;** ½ c kimchi or live-culture sauerkraut; side salad (1 c greens, ½ c other veggies) with **Lemony Dill Dressing** (4 veggies, 2 proteins, 1 grain, 1 fat)
Day 3	2 poached eggs; 1 slice whole-grain toast; 1 sliced pear (1 fruit, 1 protein, 1 grain)	1 c mixed berries; 1 serving yogurt (1 fruit, 1 protein)	**Tuna Salad with Chickpeas, Green Beans, and Tomatoes** (4 veggies, 2 proteins)	1 c cherry tomatoes dipped in **Guacamole**; 1 square dark chocolate (2 veggies, 1 fat)	**Celebration Salad;** ½ c cooked quinoa (3 veggies, 2 proteins, 1 grain, 1 fat)
Day 4	1 apple spread with 1 tbs nut butter; ½ c oatmeal made with water (1 fruit, 1 protein, 1 grain)	**Fruity Veggie Smoothie** (1 fruit, ½ veggie, 1 protein)	**Spinach and Egg Salad** (3 veggies, 2 proteins, 1 fat)	1 c sliced red peppers dipped in ½ c ricotta cheese mixed with chopped fresh thyme (2 veggies, 1 protein)	**Chicken with Peppers and Broccoli** including optional grains (2 veggies, 1 protein, 1 grain, 1 fat)
Day 5	1 c blueberries; 1 serving yogurt (1 fruit, 1 protein)	1 apple spread with 1 tbs nut butter (1 fruit, 1 protein)	**Farmer's Market Chopped Salad** (6 veggies, 1 protein, 1 fat)	30g whole-grain crackers; 30g sliced cheddar cheese (1 protein, 1 grain)	**Beef Barley Stew**; 1 square dark chocolate (2½ veggies, 2 proteins, 1 grain, 1 fat)
Day 6	**Granola Yogurt** (1 fruit, 1 protein, 1 grain)	Pear spread with 1 tbs nut butter (1 fruit, 1 protein)	**Black Bean Soup** with 30g whole-grain crackers (1½ veggies, 2 proteins, 1 grain)	1 c raw veggies dipped in **Homemade Hummus** (2 veggies, 1 protein, 1½ fat)	**Chickpeas with Tomatoes;** side salad (1 c greens, ½ c other veggies) with **Rosemary Garlic Dressing** (4½ veggies, 1 protein, 1 grain, ½ fat)
Day 7	**Baby Greens Omelette**; 1 slice whole-grain toast; 1 pear (1 fruit, 1½ veggies, 1 protein, 1 grain)	**Berry Smoothie** (1 fruit, 1 protein)	**Garlic Prawns; Summer Gazpacho** (3 veggies, 1 protein, 1½ fat)	30g cheddar cheese; 1 c cherry tomatoes dipped in **Rosemary Garlic Dressing** (2 veggies, 1 protein)	**Broccoli Asparagus Quinoa Salad;** ½ c cooked black beans; ½ c kimchi or live-culture sauerkraut (3½ veggies, 2 proteins, ½ fat)

Maintaining Your Weight Loss

The Lose Your Belly Diet is not just a weight-loss plan—it's an eating strategy that you can follow for the rest of your life.

When people follow fad diets that are impossible to stick with long-term, they stay on them just long enough to hit their weight-loss goals. Then, they ditch their crazy, unsustainable diet and go back to eating the way they did before they started losing weight.

But that's not how we roll with *The Lose Your Belly Diet*. This diet is so nutritious, so healthy, so good for you and your Little Buddies that when you reach your weight-loss goal, no big changes are needed. You simply stay on the plan, adjusting the number of daily servings of food in a way that allows you to maintain your healthy weight.

It's pretty simple: After meeting your weight goal, you can gradually add in an extra serving or two of fruits or grains per day. You eat enough to maintain your weight, but not so much that you start putting on extra pounds.

With fruits, go ahead and expand your choices beyond the prebiotic Super Fruits that you ate throughout the plan. Add in bananas, cherries, oranges, grapes, mangoes, and other enjoyable fruits. As for grains, stick with the whole grains that sustained you through your weight loss, but include an extra daily serving if you'd like.

As you add in a little more food each day, use your bathroom scale to help you determine how much more or less you can eat. If you go up a pound or two, cut back a bit on your extra fruits and grains. And if you go down a couple pounds, eat a little more.

Eventually you will find your balance and will know exactly how much to eat. That's the holy grail of weight maintenance and health: when your body and mind are in sync with how much you should eat. You may not be there right now, but it *is* possible and you *can* get there!

Eat the Same Great Foods

Although you don't have to stick exactly to the serving recommendations in Lose Your Belly EXPRESS or Lose Your Belly EXTRA, I do suggest that you keep at least some of the structure that worked for you while you were losing weight. Continue to include protein in each meal and snack. Plan on having three meals and two snacks per day to help prevent you from getting overly hungry. And although you don't have to be a slave to your measuring cups and kitchen scales, do keep a close eye on portion sizes for fats, whole grains, and protein foods so that your weight doesn't start inching up. When something works, it makes good sense to stay with it!

As for the foods you've been eating, you'll definitely want to stick with them. Keep filling your plate with the Prebiotic Superstars—vegetables and fruits— that are such an important source of fibre and nutrients for you and your Little Buddies. Continue to choose plant-based proteins more often than meats. Stick with your habit of having probiotic foods every day. The foods I recommend in *The Lose Your Belly Diet* are some of the best choices you can possibly make for the rest of your life. They're a perfect way for you to feed yourself and your Little Buddies for the long term, so there's no need to change a thing.

It will be tempting, after you reach your goal weight, to eat some of the foods that you ate regularly when you were overweight or weren't feeling your best. Listen, I'm not going to tell you that you can never have an occasional slice of birthday cake, a quarter-pound bacon burger, or an ice cream sundae. But I do urge you to limit those splurges and eat them only as a "treat" or you'll end up right back where you started.

If your weight does start to creep up again, make some adjustments right away. Cut back to one or two grains a day. Stick with two fruits daily, and lean toward Superstar Fruits such as apples, pears, and berries, which are lower in calories and higher in fibre than most other fruits. Or, you can jump right in and start following Lose Your Belly EXPRESS or EXTRA again for a week or two, or until you burn away any pounds you've added. You want to stop weight gain immediately, when the damage is minor, rather than letting the pounds add up. It's a hell of a lot easier to drop 3 pounds than it is to lose 20 pounds.

Once you get a feel for your own best maintenance strategy, weigh yourself once a week or so and make adjustments along the way. If you notice your weight has gone up, spring into action. Go back to the EXPRESS Plan if you gain four or five pounds. Or, go back to the EXTRA Plan if you gain two or three pounds. Reflect on what choices you made that led to your weight gain. Have you been eating more? Exercising less? Choosing foods that are not so great for you and your Little Buddies? Whatever it is, identify it, admit it to yourself, and create a strategy to change your behaviour while your weight gain is minor. Then, get on track and bring your weight back down.

Keep Moving

As you maintain your hard-earned weight loss, don't forget to keep moving! Exercise will help you hold on to your weight loss—and it brings so many other benefits as well. If you're finding yourself falling off the exercise bandwagon at all, go over chapter 13 and remind yourself of how important it is for you to be moving your body every day. If you haven't already bought a step counter, now may be the time to make an investment. Many people I know wear them every day because they're such a great way to remind yourself to get out there and move.

The most important suggestion I can give to you at this point is to have fun living a healthy life. Make good health your hobby! Enjoy and savour the increased energy and life force that comes with living at a healthy weight! Have a blast living an active life! Become someone who ends sentences with exclamation points!

By maintaining a healthy, active mindset, you will find so many enjoyable ways to make exercise and smart eating a part of your everyday life. Always be thinking about enjoyable physical activities you can be doing. Invite friends over to cook healthy meals filled with the delicious gut-boosting foods we've talked about in this book. Spend your Saturdays outdoors, walking, running, cycling, and enjoying gorgeous weather. Plan active vacations in which you're hiking, cycling, exploring cities, or learning new sports rather than just lying on the beach. Make it a game, rather than a chore, to hit your step count each day.

I say all this because I've seen what happens to people who don't embrace a healthy, active life. As an ER doc, I routinely spend time with chronically ill people who have not taken care of their bodies over the years. They wish more than anything that they could turn back the clock and live a better, healthier life. They would give anything for a second chance. But many of them can't. It is too late for them—but it is not too late for you. Please, don't pass up this chance.

None of us knows how long we will live. Maybe we have 50 years remaining; maybe we have a few months. Whatever it is, we owe it to ourselves to embrace and celebrate life, and one of the best ways to do that is to be as healthy and active as we can possibly be. Life is an incredible gift, and we can honour it by living every second to the absolute fullest. Make the most of your life by being active and fuelling your body in a way that best supports you (and your Little Buddies, of course). Don't be the person in the ER whose last moments are filled with nothing but regret.

This is your chance—I hope you will use it!

Learning More

The recommendations in this book are all based on our current knowledge about the human gut microbiome. But judging from how fast the field is changing—I am not kidding, new research comes out nearly every day—I'm sure that scientists will continue to uncover information about ways to help our Little Buddies. As you hear about new discoveries, I hope you'll keep a few things in mind.

First, be sceptical. Remember that if something sounds too good to be true, it probably is.

Second, be thorough. If you want to research something you've heard about, check a few different trusted sources to interpret news on microbiome developments. Some great online resources are the Mayo Clinic website (www.mayoclinic.org/patient-care-and-health-information), the Nutrition Source section of the Harvard T. H. Chan School of Public Health website (www.hsph.harvard.edu/nutritionsource/), and WebMD (http://www.webmd.com/news/). You should also check in with your doctor or healthcare provider for questions related to your own health.

Finally, stay focused on the fact that the first step in preventing health problems is to take the best possible care of your body through diet, exercise, and other healthy lifestyle choices such as not smoking, being responsible with alcohol, and following commonsense safety rules.

As Hippocrates and so many other brilliant medical practitioners have said, it's always better to prevent disease than to treat it. By taking good care of your body and following the recommendations in *The Lose Your Belly Diet*, you'll be putting yourself in a great position to prevent all kinds of health problems. That would make Hippocrates proud—and it will make me pretty happy, too.

The Lose Your Belly Diet Recipe Guide

The recipes in this guide are divided into nine sections: Breakfasts; Lunch Salads; Salad Dressings; Veggie Chow-Chows; Soups; Meatless Main Dishes; Meat, Fish, and Poultry Main Dishes; Side Dishes; and Salsas, Dips, and Spreads.

Each recipe has a Serving Tracker that lists the number of Superstar Fruits, Proteins, Grains, and Fats in each serving of the recipe.

Unless otherwise noted, when grains such as quinoa, bulgur, and barley are listed, prepare them according to their package directions and measure them *after* cooking to make sure you have the right amount.

BREAKFASTS

Berry Smoothie

Fruity Veggie Smoothie

Nutty Berry Smoothie

Granola Yogurt

Apple Walnut Breakfast Bowl

Baby Greens Omelette

Pizza Omelette

Spicy Veggie Scramble

Cheesy Mushroom Omelette

Broccoli Cheddar Breakfast Burrito

Black Bean Breakfast Bowl

Open Breakfast Sandwich

LUNCH SALADS

Spinach and Egg Salad

Tuna Salad with Chickpeas, Green Beans, and Tomatoes

Farmer's Market Chopped Salad

Cinnamon Apple Salad with Pecans

Cheese and Nut Salad

Tomato Ricotta Salad

Chicken and Avocado Salad

Green Bean Salad

SALAD DRESSINGS

Simple Vinaigrette

Lemony Dill Dressing

Lime Mint Dressing

Coriander Lime Dressing

Rosemary Garlic Dressing

Creamy Avocado Dressing

Tahini Dressing

VEGGIE CHOW-CHOWS

Summer Harvest Chow-Chow

Mediterranean Chow-Chow

Spring Greens Chow-Chow

South-of-the-Border Chow-Chow

Root Vegetable Chow-Chow

Coleslaw Chow-Chow

SOUPS

Hearty Lentil Soup

Minestrone Soup

Any Vegetable Soup

Black Bean Soup

Easy Chicken Barley Soup

Summer Gazpacho

Creamy Summer Gazpacho

MEATLESS MAIN DISHES

Loaded Veggie Burger

Quinoa-Stuffed Peppers

Bulgur with Spinach, Tomatoes, Chickpeas, and Feta Cheese

Broccoli Asparagus Quinoa Salad

Quick-Fix Spinach Lasagne

Pearl Barley with Fresh Summer Veggie Sauce

Quinoa Veggie Pilaf

Lentils with Barley and Spicy Tomato Sauce

MEAT, FISH, AND POULTRY MAIN DISHES

White Bean Chicken Chilli

Beefy-Bean Chilli

Fast and Easy Turkey Chilli

Beef Barley Stew

Celebration Salad

Chicken with Peppers and Broccoli

Pork Kebabs

Garlic Prawns

Enchiladas

Salsa Chicken

Chicken, Prawn, Beef, or Pork Stir-Fry

Baked Fish with Tomatoes and Olives

Santa Fe Pork Chops with Rice

SIDE DISHES

Bulgur Tabbouleh

Sautéed Broccoli with Garlic and Roasted Red Peppers

Roasted Root Vegetables

Salsa Beans

Rainbow Beans

Steamed Sesame Asparagus

Butterbeans with Multicoloured Peppers

Chickpeas with Tomatoes

SALSAS, DIPS, AND SPREADS

Superstar Salsa

Corn and Tomato Salsa

Homemade Hummus

Cool Cucumber Yogurt Dip

Green Goddess Dip

Rosemary-Garlic Yogurt Dip

Spinach-Onion Hummus Dip

White Bean Spread

Guacamole

Creamy Avocado White Bean Dip

Mediterranean Ricotta Dip

Greek Dip

BREAKFASTS

Berry Smoothie
(1 serving)

1 serving dairy (choose 1 of the following: 1 cup milk, 230g yogurt, 150g container of Greek yogurt, or 1 cup kefir)

1 cup frozen raspberries, blueberries, blackberries, or mixed berries

Sprinkle of spice, such as cinnamon, ginger, or nutmeg (optional)

Place all ingredients in a blender. Blend together until smooth. (If using Greek yogurt, add water if desired to adjust consistency.)

Serving Tracker:

Superstar Fruit: 1 serving

Protein: 1 serving

Fruity Veggie Smoothie
(1 serving)

1 serving dairy (choose 1 of the following: 1 cup milk, 230g yogurt, 150g container of Greek yogurt, or 1 cup kefir)

1 cup frozen raspberries, blueberries, blackberries, or mixed berries

½ cup baby spinach leaves or baby kale leaves (fresh or frozen)

1 teaspoon honey (optional until you get used to the taste of greens in your smoothie)

Sprinkle of spice, such as cinnamon, ginger, or nutmeg (optional)

Place all ingredients in a blender. Blend together until smooth. (If using Greek yogurt, add water if desired to adjust consistency.)

Serving Tracker:

Superstar Fruit: 1 serving

Superstar Veggies: ½ serving

Protein: 1 serving

Dr. T's Tasty Tip

In all smoothie recipes, if you don't love the tartness of yogurt or kefir, add in ¼ of a banana rather than using sweetened yogurt or kefir. Our goal is to help you become accustomed to less sweetness, but if you need some sweetness, bananas are a great way to add it naturally, and with a little extra fibre, too.

Nutty Berry Smoothie
(1 serving)

1 serving dairy (choose 1 of the following: 1 cup milk, 230g yogurt, 150g container of Greek yogurt, or 1 cup kefir)

1 cup frozen berries

1 tablespoon nut butter

Sprinkle of spice, such as cinnamon, ginger, or nutmeg (optional)

Place all ingredients in a blender. Blend together until smooth. (If using Greek yogurt, add water if desired to adjust consistency.)

Serving Tracker:

Superstar Fruit: 1 serving

Protein: 2 servings

Granola Yogurt
(1 serving)

1 serving yogurt (230g yogurt or 150g container of Greek yogurt)

1 cup fresh raspberries, blueberries, blackberries, or mixed berries

¼ cup granola

Sprinkle of spice, such as cinnamon, ginger, or nutmeg (optional)

In a glass bowl, spoon in yogurt and berries. Top with granola and a sprinkle of spice if using.

Serving Tracker:

Superstar Fruit: 1 serving

Protein: 1 serving

Grains: 1 serving

Apple Walnut Breakfast Bowl
(1 serving)

½ cup cottage cheese

1 apple, chopped, with skin on (1 cup)

Dash cinnamon

15g chopped walnuts

Spoon cottage cheese into a bowl. Top with apple, cinnamon, and walnuts.

Serving Tracker:

Superstar Fruit: 1 serving

Protein: 2 servings

Baby Greens Omelette
(1 serving)

Olive oil cooking spray

¼ cup white or red onion, diced

1 cup baby greens (spinach or kale leaves, chopped)

2 medium eggs

Dash of dried basil (or chopped fresh basil)

Coat a small frying pan with the olive oil cooking spray. Sauté onions and greens until veggies are soft. Scramble eggs in a glass bowl and pour over the vegetables. Sprinkle basil over egg mixture and stir slowly while cooking. Flip and cook to desired doneness.

Serving Tracker:

Superstar Veggies: 1½ servings

Protein: 1 serving

Substituting Tofu for Eggs

Although I personally don't do it, it's easy to use tofu instead of eggs in scrambled eggs. Buy firm or extra-firm tofu. Using a fork, break the tofu into small crumbles. Add them to a heated pan along with any vegetables you're using. You can also mix in a pinch of turmeric, a spice that gives tofu a yellow egg-like colour, as well as onion powder, garlic powder, herbs, or other flavours that help spice up tofu's bland taste. Cook for 5–10 minutes, or until the tofu starts to brown.

Pizza Omelette

(1 serving)

Olive oil cooking spray

¼ cup white or red onion, diced

¼ cup mushrooms, chopped

¼ cup green peppers, chopped

2 medium eggs

¼ cup passata, heated

Dash of dried basil (or chopped fresh basil)

30g mozzarella cheese, grated or sliced

Coat a small frying pan with the olive oil cooking spray. Sauté vegetables until they are soft; drain mushroom liquid if desired. Scramble eggs in a glass bowl and pour over the vegetables. Stir slowly while cooking. Flip and cook to desired doneness. Remove from heat and top with passata, basil, and mozzarella cheese. Place under the grill until cheese melts.

Serving Tracker:

Superstar Veggies: 2 servings

Protein: 2 servings

Spicy Veggie Scramble
(1 serving)

Olive oil cooking spray

¼ cup white or red onion, diced

1 cup baby spinach or baby kale, chopped

¼ cup red pepper, chopped

2 medium eggs

Small dash of chilli powder

Freshly ground black pepper

Dash of hot sauce (optional)

Coat a small frying pan with the olive oil cooking spray. Sauté vegetables until they are soft. Scramble eggs in a glass bowl, pour over the vegetables, and sprinkle with chilli powder and pepper. Stir slowly while cooking. Flip and cook to desired doneness. Season with a dash of hot sauce if desired.

Serving Tracker:

Superstar Veggies: 2 servings

Protein: 1 serving

Cheesy Mushroom Omelette
(1 serving)

Olive oil cooking spray

¼ cup white or red onion, diced

½ cup mushrooms, chopped

2 medium eggs

30g grated cheddar or other hard cheese

Freshly ground black pepper

Coat a small frying pan with the olive oil cooking spray. Sauté vegetables until they are soft; drain liquid from mushrooms if desired. Scramble eggs in a glass bowl and pour over the vegetables. Stir slowly while cooking. Flip and cook to desired doneness. Top with grated cheese and pepper, and fold one half of omelette over the other half to allow the cheese to melt.

Serving Tracker:

Superstar Veggies: 1½ servings

Protein: 2 servings

Broccoli Cheddar Breakfast Burrito
(1 serving)

Olive oil cooking spray

¼ cup white or red onion, diced

½ cup broccoli, chopped

¼ cup red pepper, chopped

2 medium eggs

1 corn tortilla

¼ cup salsa

30g grated cheddar or other hard cheese

Coat a small frying pan with the olive oil cooking spray. Sauté vegetables until they are soft. Scramble eggs in a glass bowl and pour over the vegetables. Stir slowly while cooking. Remove from heat when done. Roll egg and veggies into corn tortilla. Top with salsa and sprinkle with cheese. Place under the grill until cheese melts.

Serving Tracker:

Superstar Veggies: 2½ servings

Protein: 2 servings

Grains: 1 serving

Black Bean Breakfast Bowl
(1 serving)

Olive oil cooking spray

2 eggs

½ cup black beans, heated

½ small avocado, sliced

¼ cup salsa

Coat a small frying pan with the olive oil cooking spray. Pour in eggs, scrambling them while cooking. Place black beans in a bowl. Top with scrambled eggs, sliced avocado, and salsa.

Serving Tracker:
Superstar Veggies: ½ serving
Protein: 2 servings
Fat: 1 serving

Open Breakfast Sandwich
(1 serving)

1 slice whole-grain bread or 1 whole-grain English muffin

Olive oil cooking spray

1 medium egg

¼ cup salsa

15g grated cheddar cheese

Toast bread or English muffin. Scramble or fry egg in olive oil cooking spray. Place cooked egg on toast or muffin, top with salsa, and sprinkle with cheese. Place under the grill until cheese melts.

Serving Tracker:
Superstar Veggies: ½ serving
Protein: 1 serving
Grains: 1 serving

LUNCH SALADS

To add a dose of probiotics to any salad, mix in ½ cup of kimchi or live-culture sauerkraut per serving. Adjust salad dressing as needed.

Spinach and Egg Salad
(1 serving)

2 cups baby spinach or baby kale leaves

½ cup cherry tomatoes, sliced

2 tablespoons red onion, chopped

2 hard-boiled eggs, sliced or chopped

30g crumbled feta cheese

2 tablespoons Simple Vinaigrette (from "Dressings" section)

Combine vegetables, eggs, and cheese. Drizzle with vinaigrette.

Serving Tracker:

Superstar Veggies: 3 servings

Protein: 2 servings

Fat: 1 serving

Tuna Salad with Chickpeas, Green Beans, and Tomatoes
(1 serving)

2 cups mixed salad greens

115g canned tuna packed in water, drained

½ cup chickpeas (or other beans, such as white beans)

½ cup cooked green beans, chilled

½ cup cherry tomatoes, sliced

Fresh chopped herbs to taste

2 tablespoons Lemony Dill Dressing (from "Dressings" section)

Arrange greens on a plate. Top with tuna, chickpeas, green beans, tomatoes, and herbs. Top with dressing.

Serving Tracker:

Superstar Veggies: 4 servings

Protein: 2 servings

Farmer's Market Chopped Salad
(1 serving)

2 cups greens (spinach, romaine lettuce, rocket, or other salad greens)

2 cups raw vegetables (use whatever you pick up at the supermarket, such as tomatoes, celery, peppers, broccoli, cauliflower, corn, cabbage, cucumbers, turnips, mushrooms, onions, sugarsnap peas, radishes, summer squash, courgettes, etc.)

2 tablespoons fresh herbs (use whatever you pick up at the supermarket, such as basil, coriander, sage, thyme, mint, etc.)

½ small avocado, finely chopped

2 hard-boiled eggs, finely chopped

2 tablespoons Coriander Lime Dressing (from "Dressings" section)

Using a sharp knife, shred or chop greens, vegetables, and herbs into 1cm pieces. Combine with avocado and egg. Toss well with dressing.

Serving Tracker:

Superstar Veggies: 6 servings

Protein: 1 serving

Fat: 1 serving

Cinnamon Apple Salad with Pecans
(1 serving)

1 Granny Smith apple, diced

Dash cinnamon

2 cups romaine lettuce

Thinly sliced red onion to taste

2 tablespoons toasted pecans

2 tablespoons Simple Vinaigrette (from "Dressings" section)

Toss apple with cinnamon. Arrange romaine on a plate. Top with apples, onion, and pecans. Drizzle with vinaigrette.

Serving Tracker:
Superstar Fruits: 1 serving
Superstar Veggies: 2 servings
Protein: 1 serving
Fat: 1 serving

Cheese and Nut Salad
(1 serving)

½ cup tomato, diced

½ cup cucumber, diced

½ cup green pepper, diced

30g cheddar cheese, cubed or grated

Fresh parsley, thyme, or other herbs, chopped

2 cups salad greens, any type, chopped well

2 tablespoons Rosemary Garlic Dressing (from "Dressings" section)

2 tablespoons chopped pecans

Toss together all ingredients. Sprinkle with nuts.

Serving Tracker:
Superstar Veggies: 5 servings
Protein: 2 servings

Tomato Ricotta Salad
(1 serving)

2 cups rocket

¼ cup fresh basil

1 cup cherry tomatoes, halved

10 small olives

½ cup ricotta cheese

½ tablespoon extra-virgin olive oil

½ tablespoon balsamic vinegar

Freshly ground black pepper

Arrange the rocket, basil, tomatoes, and olives on a plate. Top with a scoop of ricotta cheese. Drizzle with oil and vinegar. Top with pepper.

Serving Tracker:
Superstar Veggies: 4½ servings
Protein: 1 serving
Fat: 1 serving

Chicken and Avocado Salad
(1 serving)

2 cups salad greens

115g cooked chicken, chopped

½ cup cooked white beans, drained

¼ cup celery, diced

1 tablespoon red onion, chopped

½ small avocado, cubed

2 tablespoons Lemony Dill Dressing (from "Dressings" section)

Place salad greens on a plate. Top with chicken, white beans, celery, red onion, and avocado. Drizzle with dressing.

Serving Tracker:
Superstar Veggies: 2½ servings
Protein: 2 servings
Fat: 1 serving

Green Bean Salad
(1 serving)

1 cup green beans, cooked and cooled

½ cup cherry tomatoes, halved

1 tablespoon fresh parsley, chopped

½ garlic clove, crushed

1 tablespoon red onion, thinly sliced

1 tablespoon olive oil

1 teaspoon cider vinegar

1 teaspoon Dijon mustard

30g flaked almonds

30g crumbled feta cheese

Combine green beans, tomatoes, parsley, garlic, and onion. In a small bowl, whisk together oil, vinegar, and mustard; toss with vegetables. Top with almonds and feta cheese.

Serving Tracker:

Superstar Veggies: 3 servings

Protein: 2 servings

Fat: 1 serving

SALAD DRESSINGS

Toss these delicious dressings with salads, or enjoy them as a dip for raw veggies.

Simple Vinaigrette
(Makes about 10 servings of 2 tablespoons each)

⅓ cup plus 2 tablespoons any kind of vinegar (balsamic, white, cider, red wine, etc.)

1 teaspoon honey

1 teaspoon lemon juice

1 teaspoon garlic (or more to taste), crushed

1 teaspoon onions or shallots (optional), minced

1 tablespoon Dijon mustard

Chopped fresh or dried herbs to taste (basil, thyme, rosemary, parsley, sage, lemongrass, coriander, etc.)

Salt and freshly ground black pepper to taste

⅔ cup extra-virgin olive oil

Whisk together vinegar, honey, lemon juice, garlic, onions or shallots if using, Dijon mustard, herbs, and salt and pepper. To create an emulsified dressing (the oil and vinegar stay combined), slowly pour olive oil into the vinegar mixture in a very thin stream while whisking vigorously. You can also use a food processor, or just combine all the ingredients in a lidded jar and shake well before using.

Serving Tracker:

Fat: 1 serving

Lemony Dill Dressing

(Makes about 8 servings of 2 tablespoons each)

1 cup plain yogurt, plain kefir, or plain drinkable yogurt

2 teaspoons extra-virgin olive oil

2 teaspoons fresh lemon juice

½ teaspoon freshly grated lemon rind

1 tablespoon fresh dill, finely chopped, or more to taste

Salt and freshly ground black pepper to taste

Combine all ingredients. Add water if needed to thin to desired consistency.

Serving Tracker:

Protein: 0 (contains a fraction of a protein serving, but we'll consider it 0)

Fat: 0 (contains a fraction of a fat serving, but we'll consider it 0)

Lime Mint Dressing

(Makes about 8 servings of 2 tablespoons each)

1 cup plain yogurt, plain kefir, or plain drinkable yogurt

2 teaspoons extra-virgin olive oil

2 teaspoons fresh lime juice

½ teaspoon freshly grated lime rind

1 tablespoon fresh mint, finely chopped, or more to taste

Salt and freshly ground black pepper to taste

Combine all ingredients. Add water if needed to thin to desired consistency.

Serving Tracker:

Protein: 0 (contains a fraction of a protein serving, but we'll consider it 0)

Fat: 0 (contains a fraction of a fat serving, but we'll consider it 0)

Coriander Lime Dressing
(Makes about 8 servings of 2 tablespoons each)

1 cup plain yogurt, plain kefir, or plain drinkable yogurt

2 teaspoons extra-virgin olive oil

2 teaspoons fresh lime juice

½ teaspoon freshly grated lime rind

1 tablespoon fresh coriander, finely chopped, or more to taste

Salt and freshly ground black pepper to taste

Combine all ingredients. Add water if needed to thin to desired consistency.

Serving Tracker:

Protein: 0 (contains a fraction of a protein serving, but we'll consider it 0)

Fat: 0 (contains a fraction of a fat serving, but we'll consider it 0)

Rosemary Garlic Dressing
(Makes about 8 servings of 2 tablespoons each)

1 cup plain yogurt, plain kefir, or plain drinkable yogurt

2 teaspoons extra-virgin olive oil

1 clove garlic, crushed

1 tablespoon fresh rosemary, finely chopped, or more to taste

1 teaspoon lemon juice

Salt and freshly ground black pepper to taste

Combine all ingredients. Add water if needed to thin to desired consistency.

Serving Tracker:

Protein: 0 (contains a fraction of a protein serving, but we'll consider it 0)

Fat: 0 (contains a fraction of a fat serving, but we'll consider it 0)

Creamy Avocado Dressing

(Makes about 8 servings of 2 tablespoons each)

1 medium avocado

1 tablespoon fresh finely chopped coriander, or more to taste

1 clove garlic

1 tablespoon olive oil

1 tablespoon fresh lime juice

½ cup plain yogurt, plain kefir, or plain drinkable yogurt

Salt and freshly ground black pepper to taste

Cut avocado in half, removing stone and scooping flesh into a blender or food processor. Add coriander, garlic, olive oil, lime juice, yogurt or kefir, salt, and pepper, and puree until smooth. Add water if needed to thin to desired consistency.

Serving Tracker:

Protein: 0 (contains a fraction of a protein serving, but we'll consider it 0)

Fat: ½ serving

Tahini Dressing

(Makes about 8 servings of 2 tablespoons each)

½ cup tahini

2 tablespoons sesame oil

1 clove garlic, crushed

1 tablespoon honey

Juice of two fresh lemons

Salt and freshly ground black pepper to taste

¼ to ½ cup of water

Whisk together tahini, sesame oil, garlic, honey, lemon juice, salt, and pepper. Whisk in enough water to thin to desired consistency.

Serving Tracker:

Fat: 1 serving

VEGGIE CHOW-CHOWS

Summer Harvest Chow-Chow

(4 servings)

4 cups summer vegetables, diced into 1cm pieces (use any combination of summer squash, courgettes, cucumber, red or orange pepper, corn, peas, asparagus, onions, radishes, etc.)

1 tablespoon oil (rapeseed, olive, or flavoured oil such as walnut or avocado)

1 tablespoon white vinegar

⅛ teaspoon salt

Freshly ground black pepper

2 tablespoons fresh dill, chopped

Place all ingredients in a large bowl. Toss well. Cover and store in the refrigerator.

Serving Tracker:

Superstar Veggies: 2 servings

Fat: 0 (contains a fraction of a fat serving, but we'll consider it 0)

Optional: Make it a light meal by adding ½ cup cooked chickpeas per serving (1 Protein).

Mediterranean Chow-Chow

(4 servings)

4 cups Mediterranean vegetables, diced into 1cm pieces (use any combination of tomatoes, garlic, onions, courgettes, fennel, mushrooms, green beans, asparagus, etc.)

1 tablespoon extra-virgin olive oil

1 tablespoon balsamic vinegar

1 teaspoon fresh lemon juice

⅛ teaspoon salt

Freshly ground black pepper

1 tablespoon fresh basil, chopped

1 tablespoon fresh oregano, chopped

Place all ingredients in a large bowl. Toss well. Cover and store in the refrigerator.

Serving Tracker:

Superstar Veggies: 2 servings

Fat: 0 (contains a fraction of a fat serving, but we'll consider it 0)

Optional: Make it a light meal by adding 30g cubed mozzarella
(1 Protein) and 10 large black olives, chopped (1 Fat), per serving.

Spring Greens Chow-Chow

(4 servings)

4 cups green vegetables, diced into 1cm pieces (use any combination of
courgettes, cucumber, green pepper, green cabbage, peas, asparagus,
spring onions, celery, green beans, etc.)

1 tablespoon rapeseed oil

1 tablespoon white vinegar

⅛ teaspoon salt

1 tablespoon fresh mint, finely chopped

1 tablespoon fresh parsley, finely chopped

Place all ingredients in a large bowl. Toss well. Cover and store in the refrigerator.

Serving Tracker:

Superstar Veggies: 2 servings

Fat: 0 (contains a fraction of a fat serving, but we'll consider it 0)

Optional: Make it a light meal by adding ½ cup cooked white beans
(1 Protein) per serving.

South-of-the-Border Chow-Chow

(4 servings)

4 cups vegetables, diced into 1cm pieces (use any combination of corn, turnips, tomatoes, garlic, red onions, peppers, chilli peppers, etc.)

1 tablespoon extra-virgin olive oil

1 tablespoon white vinegar

1 tablespoon fresh lime juice

⅛ teaspoon salt

Freshly ground black pepper

1 tablespoon fresh coriander, chopped

1 tablespoon fresh oregano, chopped

Dash chilli powder

Dash ground cumin

Optional: dash (or more) of hot sauce

Place all ingredients in a large bowl. Toss well. Cover and store in the refrigerator.

Serving Tracker:

Superstar Veggies: 2 servings

Fat: 0 (contains a fraction of a fat serving, but we'll consider it 0)

Optional: Make it a light meal by adding ½ cup cooked black beans (1 Protein) and ½ a small avocado, cubed (1 Fat) per serving.

Root Vegetable Chow-Chow
(4 servings)

4 cups root/autumn vegetables, diced into 1cm pieces (use any combination of carrots, celery, celeriac, broccoli, cauliflower, onions, red cabbage, fennel, etc.)

1 tablespoon extra-virgin olive oil

1 tablespoon cider vinegar

⅛ teaspoon salt

Freshly ground black pepper

1 tablespoon fresh thyme, chopped

1 tablespoon fresh sage, chopped

Optional: 1 pear, chopped

Place all ingredients in a large bowl. Toss well. Cover and store in the refrigerator.

Serving Tracker:

Superstar Veggies: 2 servings

Fat: 0 (contains a fraction of a fat serving, but we'll consider it 0)

Optional: Make it a light meal by adding ½ cup cooked kidney beans (1 Protein) and 30g feta cheese (1 Protein) per serving.

Coleslaw Chow-Chow
(4 servings)

4 cups traditional coleslaw vegetables, shredded or diced into 1cm pieces (use green cabbage, red cabbage, carrots, celery, celeriac, radishes, broccoli, red peppers, etc.)

1 teaspoon grated ginger root

1 tablespoon rapeseed oil

1 tablespoon cider vinegar

1 teaspoon fresh lemon juice

⅛ teaspoon salt

Freshly ground black pepper

1 tablespoon fresh parsley, chopped

1 teaspoon celery seed

Optional: 1 Granny Smith apple, chopped

Place all ingredients in a large bowl. Toss well. Cover and store in the refrigerator.

Serving Tracker:
Superstar Veggies: 2 servings
Fat: 0 (contains a fraction of a fat serving, but we'll consider it 0)
Optional: Make it a light meal by adding 115g shredded chicken (1 Protein) per serving.

SOUPS

Hearty Lentil Soup
(4 servings)

Olive oil cooking spray

1 medium onion, chopped

¾ cup celery, diced

¾ cup carrots, diced

1 garlic clove, crushed

900ml fat-free, reduced-sodium chicken, beef, or vegetable stock

450g fresh, ripe tomatoes, chopped (or 425g can chopped tomatoes with juice)

1 cup dry lentils

1 cup baby spinach, sliced thin

1 teaspoon vinegar

½ teaspoon ground cumin

1 teaspoon dried oregano

1 bay leaf

Freshly ground black pepper

Spray a saucepan or soup pot with olive oil cooking spray and heat on medium. Add onion, celery, and carrots, sautéing for a few minutes, until they start to soften. Add garlic and sauté for 1 minute. Add in all remaining ingredients. Bring to a boil. Reduce heat to low, cover, and simmer gently for 25 to 30 minutes, or until lentils are tender. Remove bay leaf before serving. If soup is thicker than you like, thin with water.

Serving Tracker:

Superstar Veggies: 1½ servings

Protein: 1 serving

Minestrone Soup

(4 servings)

900ml fat-free, reduced-sodium chicken, beef, or vegetable stock

450g fresh, ripe tomatoes, chopped (or 425g can chopped tomatoes with juice)

2 small courgettes, quartered and sliced

2 garlic cloves, crushed

1 large onion, chopped

2 stalks celery, chopped

2 carrots, sliced

2 cups canned kidney beans, drained

1 cup frozen green beans

2 teaspoons dried oregano

2 teaspoons dried basil

Parmesan cheese

In a large saucepan or soup pot, combine stock, tomatoes, courgettes, garlic, onion, celery, and carrots. Bring to a boil; cover and reduce heat. Simmer until vegetables are tender, about 20 minutes. Add kidney beans, green beans, oregano, and basil. Simmer 5–6 minutes, until green beans are tender. Top each serving with a sprinkle of Parmesan cheese prior to serving.

Serving Tracker:

Superstar Veggies: 3 servings

Protein: 1 serving

Any Vegetable Soup

(6 or more servings, depending on how many vegetables are added)

Olive oil cooking spray

1 small onion, chopped

1 garlic clove, crushed

1 cup celery, chopped

1 cup carrots, chopped

1 cup spinach or cabbage, sliced thin

½ cup (or more) of any kind of vegetable, such as green beans, wax beans, broccoli, cauliflower, mushrooms, or squash

900ml fat-free, reduced-sodium chicken, beef, or vegetable stock

450g fresh, ripe tomatoes, chopped (or 425g can chopped tomatoes with juice)

Fresh or dried parsley, basil, oregano, thyme, sage, or other herbs, to taste

Freshly ground black pepper

Spray a saucepan or soup pot with cooking spray and heat on medium. Add onion, garlic, celery, carrots, spinach, cabbage, and other vegetables. Sauté for a few minutes, stirring often, until they start to soften. Add stock, tomatoes, herbs, and pepper. Bring to a boil. Reduce heat to low, cover, and simmer for

20–30 minutes, or until the vegetables are cooked to the doneness you like. If needed, add extra stock or tomatoes.

Serving Tracker:

Superstar Veggies: 2 servings or more, depending on how many vegetables are added

---

Black Bean Soup
(4 servings)

Olive oil cooking spray

½ cup chopped red onion

2 cloves garlic, crushed

½ cup celery, chopped

½ cup carrot, chopped

1 tablespoon chilli powder (or according to taste)

1 teaspoon ground cumin

2 tablespoons fresh coriander, chopped

1½ cups reduced-sodium, fat-free chicken, beef, or vegetable stock (or more if desired)

4 cups cooked or canned black beans, drained

450g fresh, ripe tomatoes, chopped (or 425g can chopped tomatoes with juice)

Optional garnishes: chopped fresh tomatoes, chopped red onions, chopped spring onions

Spray a large saucepan or soup pot with olive oil cooking spray. Sauté onion, garlic, celery, and carrot until they begin to soften. Add in chilli powder, cumin, coriander, stock, beans, and tomatoes. Bring to a boil. Reduce heat, cover, and simmer for 15 minutes. Carefully transfer about half of the soup to a blender or food processor and process until smooth. Pour back into pot and stir well. If soup is too thick, add extra stock. Top with garnishes just before serving, or pass garnishes at table.

Serving Tracker:

Superstar Veggies: 1½ servings

Protein: 2 servings

Easy Chicken Barley Soup
(2 servings)

900ml fat-free, reduced-sodium chicken stock

½ cup carrot, sliced

½ cup celery, chopped

½ cup onion, chopped

225g cooked chicken, shredded

1 tablespoon fresh parsley, chopped

1 cup cooked pearl barley (prepared according to package directions)

Combine stock, carrots, celery, and onion in a saucepan or soup pot. Bring to a boil. Reduce heat, cover, and simmer for 20 minutes. Stir in chicken, parsley, and precooked barley. Simmer for 5 minutes.

Serving Tracker:

Superstar Veggies: 1½ servings

Protein: 1 serving

Grains: 1 serving

Summer Gazpacho
(4 servings)

1 small cucumber, peeled, seeded, and chopped

1 small red pepper, chopped

450g fresh, ripe tomatoes, chopped (or 425g can chopped tomatoes with juice)

½ small red onion, diced

2 garlic cloves, minced

1 teaspoon ground cumin

2 tablespoons fresh coriander or fresh parsley

3 cups low-sodium tomato juice or vegetable juice

Juice from 1 small lime

1 tablespoon balsamic vinegar

4 tablespoons extra-virgin olive oil

Add cucumber, pepper, tomatoes, onion, garlic, cumin, and coriander or parsley to a food processor. Puree until smooth. Add in tomato juice or vegetable juice, lime juice, vinegar, and olive oil. Mix well. Chill at least three hours or overnight. Stir well before serving. Serve in chilled bowls.

Serving Tracker:
Superstar Veggies: 3 servings
Fat: 1 serving

Creamy Summer Gazpacho
(4 servings)

Follow recipe for Summer Gazpacho, but reduce tomato juice or vegetable juice to 2 cups. Just before serving, stir in 1 cup plain, unflavoured yogurt, drinkable yogurt, or kefir.

Serving Tracker:
Superstar Veggies: 2½ servings
Protein: ¼ serving
Fat: 1 serving

MEATLESS MAIN DISHES

Some of these meatless main dishes can also serve as side dishes for meat, poultry, or fish.

Loaded Veggie Burger
(1 serving)

1 veggie burger
30g cheddar cheese
1 slice whole-grain bread or whole-grain English muffin, toasted
¼ cup guacamole
½ cup salsa

Cook veggie burger according to package directions. Melt cheese on top. Place on toast or English muffin. Top with guacamole and salsa.

Serving Tracker:

Superstar Veggies: 1 serving

Protein: 2 servings

Grains: 1 serving

Fat: 1 serving

Quinoa-Stuffed Peppers
(4 servings)

4 red peppers, cut in half from top to bottom, seeds, membranes, and stem removed

Freshly ground black pepper

1 small orange pepper, well chopped

1 small green pepper, well chopped

1 onion, chopped

2 tablespoons extra-virgin olive oil

450g fresh, ripe tomatoes, chopped (or 425g can chopped tomatoes with juice)

½ cup *uncooked* quinoa

1 tablespoon Worcestershire sauce

1 teaspoon chilli powder (or according to taste)

1 teaspoon ground cumin

1 cup passata

1 cup grated cheddar cheese

Preheat oven to 190°C. Bring a large pot of water to boil. Immerse red peppers in boiling water for 3 minutes. Drain peppers and discard water. Arrange peppers, open-side up, in a large glass baking dish. Sprinkle with black pepper. In a large pan, sauté chopped orange and green peppers and onion in olive oil until vegetables begin to soften. Add in tomatoes, quinoa, Worcestershire sauce, chilli powder, cumin, half of the passata, and 1 cup water. Mix well. Bring to a boil. Reduce heat to low, cover, and simmer

15 minutes, or until quinoa is cooked. Stir half the cheese into the quinoa mixture and mix well. Spoon the quinoa-cheese mixture into the cavities of the red peppers in the baking dish. Pour the remaining passata over all. Top with remaining cheese. Bake 15–20 minutes, or until bubbly.

Serving Tracker:

Superstar Veggies: 4 servings

Protein: 1 serving

Grains: 1 serving

Fat: ½ serving

Bulgur with Spinach, Tomatoes, White Beans, and Feta Cheese
(4 servings)

½ cup chopped onions

3 cups fresh spinach, chopped well

1–2 garlic cloves, crushed

2 tablespoons extra-virgin olive oil

1 cup chopped fresh tomatoes or 1 cup canned chopped tomatoes with juice

½ teaspoon allspice

½ teaspoon ground cumin

½ teaspoon cinnamon

Dash of salt

Freshly ground pepper

2 cups cooked or canned white beans, drained

2 cups cooked bulgur (prepared according to package directions and kept warm)

115g crumbled feta cheese

In a large frying pan, sauté onions, spinach, and garlic in olive oil until they start to soften. Stir in tomatoes, allspice, cumin, cinnamon, salt, and pepper, and cook for 2–3 minutes. Stir in white beans and bulgur; mix well while heating through. Remove from heat and sprinkle with feta cheese.

Serving Tracker:

Superstar Veggies: 1½ servings

Protein: 2 servings

Grains: 1 serving

Fat: 1 serving

Broccoli Asparagus Quinoa Salad
(4 servings)

Dressing:

2 tablespoons olive oil

2 tablespoons rice or cider vinegar

2 teaspoons Dijon mustard

1 garlic clove, crushed

Salt and pepper to taste

Zest of one orange

2 tablespoons fresh orange juice

Salad:

2 cups cooked and cooled quinoa (prepared according to package directions) or use frozen cooked quinoa

½ cup chopped red, yellow, or orange pepper, or a combination

½ cup chopped red onion

½ cup broccoli, cut into small pieces

½ cup asparagus, cut into small pieces

¼ cup fresh parsley, chopped (or coriander, mint, thyme, or other fresh herbs)

8 cups salad greens, such as romaine lettuce or mixed greens

½ cup chopped cashews or pecans

Make dressing by combining ingredients and mixing well. Make salad by mixing all ingredients except salad greens and nuts. Toss quinoa-vegetable mixture with half of the dressing, mixing well. Toss greens with the other half of the dressing. Divide greens into four bowls or plates. Top with quinoa salad. Sprinkle with nuts.

Serving Tracker:

Superstar Veggies: 3 servings

Protein: 1 serving

Grains: 1 serving

Fat: ½ serving

Quick-Fix Spinach Lasagne

If you remember this dish from my book The Doctor's Diet, *you're right—it's one of my favourites!*

(4 servings)

450g low-fat cottage cheese

1 bag (280g) fresh spinach

1 egg

1 teaspoon chilli flakes

Freshly ground black pepper to taste

Olive oil cooking spray

225g whole-wheat lasagne sheets, uncooked

1 cup homemade or bought passata

½ cup grated mozzarella cheese

Preheat oven to 175°C. In a bowl, combine cottage cheese, spinach, egg, and red and black pepper. Spritz a baking dish with cooking spray. Spread out half the lasagne sheets. Cover with the cheese/spinach filling; top with the remaining sheets. Pour passata over the sheets; sprinkle with mozzarella cheese. Bake for 45–50 minutes.

Serving Tracker:

Superstar Veggies: 3 servings

Protein: 2 servings

Grains: 2 servings

Pearl Barley with Fresh Summer Veggie Sauce
(4 servings)

1 onion, chopped

1 clove garlic, diced

2 tablespoons olive oil

1 small courgettes, chopped into 1cm pieces

1 small summer squash, chopped into 1cm pieces

1 red pepper, chopped into 1cm pieces

1 cup fresh mushrooms, sliced

2–3 fresh tomatoes, chopped, or 2 cups cherry tomatoes, halved

1 tablespoon dried oregano

½ cup white wine

Dash salt

Freshly ground black pepper

1–2 tablespoons tomato paste (optional if you like a thicker sauce)

2 cups cooked barley (prepared according to package directions and kept hot)

115g grated mozzarella cheese

Fresh basil cut in thin ribbons

In a large frying pan, sauté onion and garlic in olive oil over medium heat until slightly softened. Add in the courgette, summer squash, red peppers, and mushrooms; sauté for about 5 minutes. Add in tomatoes, oregano, white wine, salt, and pepper. Bring to a boil, then simmer gently, covered, for about 10–15 minutes, or until tomatoes fall apart. Stir in tomato paste, if using. Spoon the sauce over hot barley. Top with mozzarella cheese and fresh basil.

Serving Tracker:

Superstar Veggies: 3½ servings

Protein: 1 serving

Grains: 1 serving

Fat: ½ serving

Quinoa Veggie Pilaf
(4 servings)

½ cup carrots, chopped

½ cup celery, chopped

½ cup spring onion, chopped

½ cup green pepper, chopped

½ cup red pepper, chopped

½ garlic cloves, crushed

2 tablespoons extra-virgin olive oil

1 tablespoon fresh or dried parsley

Dash of salt

Freshly ground black pepper

2 cups cooked quinoa (prepared according to package directions and kept warm; or use frozen cooked quinoa)

1 cup almonds, flaked or chopped

In a large frying pan, sauté vegetables and garlic in olive oil until they start to soften. Stir in parsley, salt, and pepper, and cook for one minute longer. Stir in cooked quinoa; mix well while heating through. Remove from heat and sprinkle with almonds.

Serving Tracker:

Superstar Veggies: 1 serving

Protein: 2 servings

Grains: 1 serving

Fat: ½ serving

Lentils with Barley and Spicy Tomato Sauce
(4 servings)

2 garlic cloves, crushed

1 onion, chopped

2 tablespoons olive oil

1 teaspoon dried oregano

1 teaspoon dried basil

450g fresh, ripe tomatoes, chopped (or 425g can chopped tomatoes with juice)

1 cup passata

½ teaspoon chilli flakes (or more to taste)

2 cups cooked or canned and drained lentils

2 cups cooked pearl barley (prepared according to package directions and kept warm)

In a large saucepan, sauté garlic and onion in olive oil until soft. Add in oregano, basil, tomatoes, passata, and chilli flakes. Bring to a boil, then cover and simmer 15 minutes. Stir in lentils and barley, and heat through.

Serving Tracker:

Superstar Veggies: 2 servings

Protein: 1 serving

Grains: 1 serving

MEAT, FISH, AND POULTRY MAIN DISHES

White Bean Chicken Chilli
(4 servings)

2 tablespoons extra-virgin olive oil

450g skinless chicken breast, cut into bite-size pieces

1 onion, peeled and diced

1–2 garlic cloves, crushed

1 red pepper, diced

1 jalapeño pepper, seeded and diced (or use seeds for extra heat)

450g fresh, ripe tomatoes, chopped (or 425g can chopped tomatoes with juice)

1 cup passata

1 tablespoon chilli powder (or according to taste)

1 teaspoon ground cumin

2 teaspoons oregano

¼ teaspoon cayenne pepper

½ cup diced mild green chillies (or according to taste)

2 cups cooked or canned white beans, drained

1 small avocado, cubed

Optional garnishes: fresh salsa or chopped fresh tomatoes, chopped red or spring onions

Add olive oil to a large saucepan and heat on medium. Sauté chicken until cooked through. Remove to a plate and set aside. Add onion, garlic, red pepper, and jalapeño to oil and sauté a few minutes, until tender. Add chicken back into saucepan, along with tomatoes, passata, chilli powder, cumin, oregano, cayenne pepper, green chillies, and beans. Bring to a boil, and then simmer 20 minutes. Top with avocado cubes. Add optional garnishes just before serving, or pass at table.

Serving Tracker:
Superstar Veggies: 2½ servings, plus garnishes
Protein: 2 servings
Fat: 1 serving

Beefy-Bean Chilli
(4 servings)

Olive oil cooking spray

225g lean minced beef

1 large onion, chopped

2–3 garlic cloves, crushed

1 tablespoon chilli powder (or according to taste)

1 teaspoon ground cumin

2 teaspoons oregano

¼ teaspoon cayenne pepper

450g fresh, ripe tomatoes, chopped (or 425g can chopped tomatoes with juice)

2 cups passata (or more for saucier chilli)

2 cups kidney beans

Optional garnishes: fresh salsa or chopped fresh tomatoes, chopped red or spring onions

Spray a large saucepan with cooking spray and heat on medium. Add minced beef and sauté until mostly cooked, breaking beef up while cooking. Drain fat. Add onion and garlic, and sauté for 2–3 minutes, or until they start to soften. Add in chilli powder, cumin, oregano, cayenne pepper, tomatoes, passata, and beans. Bring to a boil. Reduce heat, cover, and simmer for 20 minutes. Top with garnishes just before serving, or pass garnishes at table.

Serving Tracker:

Superstar Veggies: 2½ servings

Protein: 2 servings

Fast and Easy Turkey Chilli
(4 servings)

450g minced turkey breast

2 cups black beans, cooked or canned and drained

1 tablespoon chilli powder (or according to taste)

6 cups salsa, homemade or from a jar

In a large nonstick frying pan or saucepan, sauté turkey until browned. Drain fat. Add in beans, chilli powder, and salsa. Bring to a boil. Reduce heat, cover, and simmer for 15 minutes.

Serving Tracker:

Superstar Veggies: 3 servings

Protein: 2 servings

Beef Barley Stew
(4 servings)

450g boneless sirloin, cut into 2.5cm cubes

1 medium onion, diced

470ml passata

1 cup fat-free, reduced-sodium chicken, beef, or vegetable stock

1 tablespoon Worcestershire sauce

4 medium carrots, sliced

4 celery stalks, sliced

225g fresh green beans, chopped

1 dried bay leaf

Fresh or dried herbs, to taste, such as parsley, thyme, rosemary, or marjoram

2 cups cooked pearl barley (prepared according to package directions)

Combine all ingredients except herbs and barley in a large pot. Bring to a boil. Cover and simmer on very low heat for 1 hour, stirring occasionally. Add herbs for the last 5 minutes of cooking. Remove bay leaf. Mix cooked pearl barley into stew just before serving.

Serving Tracker:

Superstar Veggies: 2½ servings

Protein: 2 servings

Grains: 1 serving

Celebration Salad
(4 servings)

2 cups sweet potato, cubed and peeled

1 spring onion, chopped

½ cup celery, chopped

½ cup red pepper, chopped

½ cup cucumbers, chopped

¼ cup fresh parsley, chopped

¼ cup extra-virgin olive oil

2 tablespoons cider vinegar

2 tablespoons Dijon mustard

1 tablespoon honey

340–450g baked, roasted, or grilled turkey, cut into cubes

55g walnuts

2 tablespoons dried cranberries

4 cups salad greens

In a saucepan, boil sweet potatoes in water until just tender, about 6–8 minutes. Drain and cool completely. Combine sweet potatoes with onion, celery, red pepper, cucumbers, and parsley. Make dressing by whisking together olive oil, vinegar, mustard, and honey. Toss salad with dressing. Top with turkey. Sprinkle with walnuts and dried cranberries. Serve over salad greens.

Serving Tracker:

Superstar Veggies: 3 servings

Protein: 2 servings

Fat: 1 serving

Chicken with Peppers and Broccoli
(4 servings)

450g skinless chicken breast, cut into bite-size pieces

2 tablespoons grated ginger root

2 garlic cloves, crushed (optional)

2 tablespoons extra-virgin olive oil

2 cups peppers, any colours, cut into matchsticks

2 cups fresh broccoli florets (optional)

2 tablespoons low-sodium soy sauce

2 tablespoons rice vinegar

2 tablespoons sesame oil

1 tablespoon mild chilli paste

Optional: 2 cups cooked grains (quinoa, brown rice, etc.)

In a large frying pan, sauté chicken, ginger, and garlic in olive oil until chicken is cooked through. Remove chicken from pan. Add peppers and broccoli in pan and sauté until tender. Add chicken back into pan. In a small bowl, whisk together soy sauce, vinegar, sesame oil, and chilli paste. Toss sauce with chicken and vegetables. Serve over brown rice or other grain, if using.

Serving Tracker:

Superstar Veggies: 2 servings

Protein: 1 serving

Grains: 1 serving (if using grains)

Fat: 1 serving

Pork Kebabs
(4 servings)

450g boneless loin pork chops, cut into 2.5cm cubes

1 medium red pepper, cut into bite-size pieces

1 medium green pepper, cut into bite-size pieces

1 red onion, cut into 2.5cm pieces

1 tablespoon sesame oil

1 tablespoon soy sauce

Freshly ground black pepper

Thread pork, pepper chunks, and red onion on kebab skewers. Mix sesame oil and soy sauce; brush onto skewers. Sprinkle with black pepper. Grill under a medium heat until pork is cooked through, approximately 8–12 minutes.

Serving Tracker:

Superstar Veggies: 1½ servings

Protein: 2 servings

Fat: 0 (contains a fraction of a fat serving, but we'll consider it 0)

Garlic Prawns
(4 servings)

450g large uncooked prawns, shelled and deveined

2 garlic cloves, crushed

2 tablespoons extra-virgin olive oil

1 tablespoon honey

¼ cup dry white wine

In a frying pan, sauté prawns and garlic in olive oil until they are cooked. Add honey and wine. Simmer for 1–2 minutes.

Serving Tracker:

Protein: 1 serving

Fat: ½ serving

Enchiladas
(4 servings)

Enchilada sauce:

1 onion, finely chopped

2 cloves garlic, crushed

1 tablespoon extra-virgin olive oil

2 tablespoons chilli powder without salt (or according to taste)

1 tablespoon ground cumin

½ cup fat-free, reduced-sodium chicken, beef or vegetable stock

2 cups passata

Enchiladas:

1 onion, chopped

1 tablespoon extra-virgin olive oil

225g minced beef, turkey, or chicken

1 cup cooked or canned black beans, drained

2 cups cooked brown rice

55g grated Monterey Jack cheese

To make enchilada sauce: Sauté onions and garlic in olive oil until onions are translucent. Mix in spices and cook 1 minute. Stir in stock and passata, bring to a boil, cover, and simmer over low heat for 10 minutes.

To make enchiladas: In a large frying pan, sauté onions in olive oil until soft. Add minced meat and sauté until browned. Add enchilada sauce and beans. Bring to a boil, reduce heat, cover, and simmer over low heat for 5–10 minutes. Serve over brown rice; top with grated cheese.

Serving Tracker:

Superstar Veggies: 1½ servings

Protein: 2 servings

Grains: 1 serving

Fat: 1 serving

Salsa Chicken
(4 servings)

1 cup salsa, homemade or from a jar

1 teaspoon ground cumin

1 teaspoon chilli powder (or according to taste)

1 tablespoon fresh lime juice

450g skinless, boneless chicken breasts

Olive oil cooking spray

Fresh coriander, chopped

Preheat oven to 190°C. In a bowl, combine salsa, cumin, chilli powder, and fresh lime juice. Place chicken in a baking dish that has been sprayed with olive oil cooking spray. Pour salsa mixture over chicken, flipping chicken until well coated with salsa. Bake 20–30 minutes, or until chicken is cooked through. During cooking, baste chicken occasionally with salsa. Top with fresh coriander.

Serving Tracker:

Superstar Veggies: ½ serving

Protein: 1 serving

Chicken, Prawn, Beef, or Pork Stir-Fry
(4 servings)

2 tablespoons rapeseed oil, divided

450g chicken OR 450g prawns OR 230–350g beef sirloin or pork loin, cut into bite-size pieces

1 cup red pepper, cut in 2.5cm strips

1 cup yellow pepper, cut in 2.5cm strips

1 cup cauliflower florets, cut in 2.5cm strips

1 cup broccoli florets, chopped

1 cup celery stalks, chopped

1 cup bean sprouts

½ cup fat-free, reduced-sodium chicken, beef, or vegetable stock

2 tablespoons low-sodium soy sauce

1 tablespoon chilli paste (or according to taste)

½ cup peanuts or almonds

Optional: 2 cups cooked whole grains (brown rice, quinoa, pearl barley, etc.)

Heat 1 tablespoon of the oil in a wok or frying pan. Stir-fry chicken, prawns, beef, or pork until cooked through. Turn off heat and remove to a plate. Add remaining 1 tablespoon of oil to pan. Over medium heat, stir-fry peppers, cauliflower, broccoli, celery, and sprouts. Cook until crisp-tender. Combine stock, soy sauce, and chilli paste; stir into vegetables, add meat back into pan, and heat for 2–3 minutes. Sprinkle with nuts. Serve over whole grains, if using.

Serving Tracker:

Superstar Veggies: 3 servings

Protein: 2 servings

Grains: 1 serving (if using optional whole grains)

Fat: 1 serving

Baked Fish with Tomatoes and Olives
(4 servings)

450g cod, flounder or other white fish (4 fillets)

1 tablespoon extra-virgin olive oil

3 plum tomatoes, thinly sliced

2 garlic cloves, crushed

1 teaspoon dried oregano

20 small olives, sliced

Preheat oven to 200°C. Brush both sides of the fish fillets with olive oil. Place them in a glass baking dish. Top with tomato slices; sprinkle with garlic, oregano, and olives. Bake for 15–20 minutes, or until fish flakes easily with a fork.

Serving Tracker:

Superstar Veggies: ½ serving

Protein: 1 serving

Fat: ½ serving

Santa Fe Pork Chops with Rice

(4 servings)

450g boneless pork chops

1 teaspoon ground cumin

1 teaspoon oregano

2 tablespoons extra-virgin olive oil

1 onion, chopped

1 red pepper, chopped

2 garlic cloves, crushed

450g fresh, ripe tomatoes, chopped (or 425g chopped tomatoes with juice)

2 teaspoons Worcestershire sauce

½ cup chopped green chillies (or according to taste)

½ teaspoon chilli flakes

115g grated Monterey Jack cheese

2 cups cooked brown rice

Sprinkle pork chops with cumin and oregano, pressing them into the pork. In a large frying pan, brown pork chops in oil. Remove to a plate when cooked. Add onions, pepper, and garlic to pan and sauté until soft. Add tomatoes, Worcestershire sauce, green chillies, and chilli flakes to pan. Bring to a boil, then reduce heat to very low. Add pork chops to pan, spooning sauce and vegetables over pork. Cover and simmer for 20 minutes. Sprinkle with grated cheese and allow to melt before serving. Serve over brown rice.

Serving Tracker:

Superstar Veggies: 2 servings

Protein: 3 servings

Fat: ½ serving

Grains: 1 serving

SIDE DISHES

Most of these side dishes make great lunches as well. Have them as is or boost their protein content by tossing in some leftover fish, shellfish, chicken, tofu, or sliced hard-boiled eggs.

Bulgur Tabbouleh
(4 servings)

2 cups cooked bulgur (prepared according to package directions and cooled)

1 cup tomatoes, chopped

1 cup cucumber, chopped

4 spring onions, finely chopped

1 bunch fresh parsley, finely chopped

¼ cup fresh mint leaves, finely chopped

2 cloves garlic, finely chopped

Juice of 1 lemon

4 tablespoons extra-virgin olive oil

Combine all ingredients and mix well.

Serving Tracker:

Superstar Veggies: 1 serving

Grains: 1 serving

Fat: 1 serving

Sautéed Broccoli with Garlic and Roasted Red Peppers
(4 servings)

1–2 garlic cloves, crushed

2 tablespoons olive oil

4 cups broccoli florets, cut into bite-size pieces

½ cup roasted red peppers from a jar, drained and diced

In a large frying pan, sauté garlic in olive oil over medium heat for 1–2 minutes. Add broccoli and sauté until crisp-tender. Stir in roasted red peppers.

Serving Tracker:

Superstar Veggies: 2 servings

Fat: ½ serving

Roasted Root Vegetables
(4 servings)

6 cups chopped or sliced root vegetables (any combination of carrots, sweet potatoes, red onions, parsnips, celeriac, swede, leeks)

2 tablespoons extra-virgin olive oil

1 tablespoon dry or 2 tablespoons fresh chopped herbs (or more to taste), such as rosemary, thyme, sage, or parsley

¼ teaspoon salt

Freshly ground black pepper

Preheat oven to 200°C. Place all vegetables in a plastic bag. Add in oil, herbs, salt, and pepper, and seal bag. Shake bag to distribute oil and herbs evenly. Pour onto a large baking tray. Roast in oven for 30–45 minutes.

Serving Tracker:

Superstar Veggies: 3 servings

Fat: ½ serving

Salsa Beans
(4 servings)

2 cups cooked or canned and drained black beans, kidney beans, or other beans

1 cup salsa, homemade or from jar

½ teaspoon ground cumin

½ teaspoon chilli powder (or according to taste)

Combine beans, salsa, and spices in a saucepan and heat until warm.

Serving Tracker:

Superstar Veggies: ½ serving

Protein: 1 serving

Rainbow Beans
(4 servings)

½ cup *each* of FOUR different kinds of beans, such as black beans, kidney beans, white beans, aduki beans, chickpeas, or other beans, cooked or canned and drained

1 cup fresh or frozen green beans, cooked, cooled, and chopped

1 cup fresh or frozen wax beans, cooked, cooled and chopped

1 cup orange pepper, chopped

1 cup red pepper, chopped

½ cup red onion, finely chopped

1–2 garlic cloves, crushed

2 tablespoons extra-virgin olive oil

2 tablespoons red wine vinegar

¼ cup fresh parsley, fresh dill, or fresh thyme, chopped

Combine all ingredients. Serve chilled or at room temperature

Serving Tracker:
Superstar Veggies: 2 servings
Protein: 1 serving
Fat: ½ serving

Steamed Sesame Asparagus
(2 servings)

450g asparagus spears, trimmed

1 tablespoon toasted sesame oil

Dash of salt

Freshly ground black pepper

2 tablespoons toasted sesame seeds

Steam asparagus until slightly tender (3–5 minutes for thinner stalks; 5–7 minutes for thicker stalks). Remove from heat. Toss with oil, salt, and pepper. Sprinkle with sesame seeds.

Serving Tracker:

Superstar Veggies: 1 serving

Fat: 1 serving

Butterbeans with Multicoloured Peppers
(4 servings)

2 cups peppers (any combination of red, yellow, orange, and green), chopped

2 tablespoons extra-virgin olive oil

2 cups butterbeans (cooked according to package directions)

½ teaspoon ground cumin

2 tablespoons chopped fresh parsley

Sauté peppers in olive oil until tender. Add butterbeans, cumin, and parsley, and sauté until heated through.

Serving Tracker:

Superstar Veggies: 2 servings

Fat: ½ serving

Chickpeas with Tomatoes
(2 servings)

1 cup canned chickpeas, drained

½ cup cucumber, chopped

2 tablespoons red onion, chopped

1 teaspoon garlic, crushed

2 cups cherry tomatoes, halved

1 tablespoon olive oil

1 tablespoon balsamic vinegar

Fresh chopped parsley to taste

Dash of pepper

Toss all ingredients together.

Serving Tracker:

Superstar Veggies: 2½ servings

Protein: 1 serving

Fat: ½ serving

SALSAS, DIPS, AND SPREADS

People tend to eat way more raw veggies when they have something fabulous to dip them in. Serve these salsas, dips, and spreads with a big platter of raw veggies, and watch them all disappear.

Superstar Salsa
(4 large servings)

2 425g cans chopped tomatoes OR 900g ripe fresh tomatoes

1 medium onion, brown or red, chopped

2–4 garlic cloves, crushed

Juice of 2 small limes

Dash of salt

1 jalapeño pepper, seeds removed, finely chopped (or use some seeds for extra heat)

¼ cup chopped fresh coriander (or more to taste)

If using canned tomatoes, drain some or all of the juice, if desired. If using fresh tomatoes, chop into 1cm pieces; drain some or all of the juice if desired. Combine all ingredients in a bowl and mix gently.

Serving Tracker:

Superstar Veggies: 2 servings

Corn and Tomato Salsa
(2 servings)

450g fresh, ripe tomatoes (or 425g can chopped tomatoes)

½ cup red onion, chopped

½ garlic cloves, crushed

1 cup fresh baby corn kernels (or frozen and thawed)

½ jalapeño pepper, seeds removed, finely chopped (or use some seeds
   for extra heat)

2 tablespoons chopped fresh coriander (or more to taste)

Juice of 1 small lime

Dash of salt

If using canned tomatoes, drain some or all of the juice, if desired. If using fresh tomatoes, chop into 1cm pieces; drain some or all of the juice if desired. Combine all ingredients in a bowl and mix gently.

Serving Tracker:

Superstar Veggies: 1½ servings

Homemade Hummus
(4 servings)

2 cups canned chickpeas, drained

¼ cup extra-virgin olive oil

2 cloves garlic, crushed

2 tablespoons tahini

1 teaspoon ground cumin

Juice of 1 lemon

Fresh parsley, chopped

Put everything but the parsley in a food processor and process until smooth. Sprinkle with parsley before serving.

Serving Tracker:

Protein: 1 serving

Fat: 1½ servings

Cool Cucumber Yogurt Dip
(4 servings)

2 containers (140–170g) plain Greek yogurt

½ small cucumber, chopped into very small pieces

1 garlic clove, crushed

2 tablespoons fresh lemon juice

2 tablespoons fresh dill or fresh mint, finely chopped

Dash of cayenne pepper

Combine all ingredients and mix well.

Serving Tracker:

Protein: ½ serving

Green Goddess Dip
(2 servings)

2 tablespoons extra-virgin olive oil

2 cloves garlic, crushed

½ cup fresh basil

½ cup fresh parsley or fresh coriander

1 tablespoon fresh lemon juice

1 container (140–170g) plain Greek yogurt

1 spring onion, finely chopped

Combine all ingredients except yogurt and spring onion in a blender or food processor. Blend/process until smooth. Mix into yogurt. Sprinkle with spring onion. Serve with raw vegetables for dipping.

Serving Tracker:

Fat: 1 serving

Protein: ½ serving

Rosemary-Garlic Yogurt Dip
(2 servings)

2 garlic cloves, crushed (or more to taste)

1 teaspoon fresh or dried rosemary leaves, chopped fine (or more to taste)

1 container (140–170g) Greek yogurt

Combine all ingredients.

Serving Tracker:

Protein: ½ serving

Spinach-Onion Hummus Dip

(4 servings)

2 cups fresh spinach

2 cups canned chickpeas, drained

¼ cup extra-virgin olive oil

2 cloves garlic, crushed

2 tablespoons tahini

Juice of 1 lemon

2 tablespoons fresh chives, chopped

Put everything but the chives in a food processor and process until smooth. Sprinkle with chives before serving.

Serving Tracker:

Superstar Veggies: ½ serving

Protein: 1 serving

Fat: 1½ servings

White Bean Spread

(4 servings)

450g can white beans, drained

2 garlic cloves

2 tablespoons olive oil

1 tablespoon plus 1 teaspoon fresh finely chopped herbs, separated (use parsley, rosemary, thyme, coriander, basil, or any other fresh herbs)

1 teaspoon fresh lemon juice

Combine all ingredients except the 1 teaspoon chopped fresh herbs in a food processor. Process until creamy. Spoon into a bowl; sprinkle with remaining herbs.

Serving Tracker:

Protein: 1 serving

Fat: ½ serving

Guacamole
(4 servings)

2 small avocados, ripe

1 teaspoon lime juice

¼ cup red onion, diced

¼ jalapeño pepper with seeds, finely chopped (optional)

½ cup chopped tomato

1 tablespoon fresh coriander, chopped

1 garlic clove, crushed

Dash of salt

Cut avocados in half, remove stone, and scoop flesh into a bowl. Mash with a potato masher or fork. Mix in lime juice, red onion, jalapeño (if using), tomato, coriander, garlic, and salt. Stir well.

Serving Tracker:

Fat: 1 serving

Creamy Avocado White Bean Dip
(4 servings)

2 small avocados, ripe

½ cup cooked or canned white beans, drained

1 container (140–170g) plain Greek yogurt

1 teaspoon lime juice

¼ cup red onion, diced

¼ jalapeño pepper with seeds, finely chopped (optional)

½ cup chopped tomato

1 tablespoon fresh coriander, chopped, plus extra for garnish

1 garlic clove, crushed

Dash of salt

Cut avocados in half, remove stone, and scoop flesh into a bowl. Mash with a potato masher or fork. In a separate bowl, mash beans with a potato masher or fork. Combine avocado, beans, and yogurt. Mix in lime juice, red onion, jalapeño (if using), tomato, coriander, garlic, and salt. Stir well. Garnish with coriander before serving.

Serving Tracker:

Fat: 1 serving

Protein: ½ serving

Mediterranean Ricotta Dip
(2 servings)

1 cup ricotta cheese

1 tablespoon fresh basil, chopped well

1 clove garlic, crushed

2 tablespoons extra-virgin olive oil, separated

Dash of salt

Freshly ground black pepper

Combine ricotta, basil, garlic, 1½ tablespoon oil, salt, and pepper. Place in serving bowl. Drizzle with remaining ½ tablespoon of olive oil.

Serving Tracker:

Fat: 1 serving

Protein: 1 serving

Greek Dip
(2 servings)

1 cup chickpeas, drained

2 tablespoons olive oil

2 tablespoons fresh oregano, finely chopped

10 large black olives, chopped

Mash chickpeas with a fork. Add olive oil and oregano and mix well. Top with black olives.

Serving Tracker:

Fat: 1½ servings

Protein: 1 serving

Bibliography

Introduction: Your Gut Health/Weight Loss Opportunity

David, L. A., et al. "Diet Rapidly and Reproducibly Alters the Human Gut Microbiome." *Nature* 505, no. 7484 (January 2014): 559–563. http://www.nature.com/nature/journal/v505/n7484/full/nature12820.html.

Chapter 1: Meet the Microbes

American Microbiome Institute. "Cigarette Smoke Changes the Gut Microbiome." http://www.microbiomeinstitute.org/blog/2015/6/11/cigarette-smoke-changes-the-gut-microbiome.

Center for Ecogenetics and Environmental Health, University of Washington, "Fast Facts About the Human Microbiome." http://depts.washington.edu/ceeh/downloads/FF_Microbiome.pdf.

Clarke, Siobahn F. et al. "Exercise and Associated Dietary Extremes Impact on Gut Microbial Diversity." *Gut* 63, no. 12 (December 2014): 1913–20. http://gut.bmj.com/content/early/2014/04/29/gutjnl-2013-306541.abstract%20?version=meter+at+11&module=meter-Links&pgtype=Blogs&contentId=&mediaId=%25%25ADID%25%25&referrer=https%3A%2F%2Fwww.google.com&priority=true&action=click&contentCollection=meter-links-click.

D'Argenio, V., and F. Salvatore. "The Role of the Gut Microbiome in the Healthy Adult Status." *Clinica Chimica Acta* 451 (2015): 97–102. http://www.sciencedirect.com/science/article/pii/S0009898115000170.

Khanna, S., and P. K. Tosh. "A Clinician's Primer on the Role of the Microbiome in Human Health and Disease." *Mayo Clinic Proceedings* 89, no. 1 (January 2014): 107–114. http://www.mayoclinicproceedings.org/article/S0025-6196%2813%2900886-0/pdf.

Kohn, David. "Joint Pain, From the Gut," *Atlantic*, January 12, 2015. http://www.theatlantic.com/health/archive/2015/01/joint-pain-from-the-gut/383772/.

Mutlu, E. A. et al. "Colonic Microbiome is Altered in Alcoholism." *American Journal of Physiology Gastrointestinal and Liver Physiology* 302, no. 9 (May 2012): G966–G978. http://ajpgi.physiology.org/content/302/9/G966.

National Institutes of Health. "Human Microbiome Project." https://commonfund.nih .gov/hmp/overview.

Chapter 2: Your Very Busy Buddies

Center for Ecogenetics and Environmental Health, University of Washington. "Fast Facts About the Human Microbiome." http://depts.washington.edu/ceeh/downloads /FF_Microbiome.pdf.

Centers for Disease Control and Prevention. "Healthcare-Associated Infections." https://www.cdc.gov/hai/organisms/cdiff/cdiff_infect.html.

Openbiome. "What is Faecal Transplantation?" http://www.openbiome.org/about-fmt.

Youngster, I. et al. "Oral, Capsulized, Frozen Faecal Microbiota Transplantation for Relapsing Clostridium difficile Infection." *Journal of the American Medical Association* 312, no. 17 (November 5, 2014): 1772–1778. http://jama.jamanetwork.com/article .aspx?articleid=1916296.

Chapter 3: Microbiome Balance and Weight Gain

Goodrich, J. K. et al. "Human Genetics Shape the Gut Microbiome." *Cell* 159 (November 6, 2014): 789–799. http://ac.els-cdn.com/S0092867414012410 /1-s2.0-S0092867414012410-main.pdf?_tid=e10913fa-2db0-11e6-ae98 -00000aab0f6c&acdnat=1465415019_ba372cc5e98b6c9ac608e61994c37c98.

Ridaura, Vanessa K. et al. "Gut Microbiota from Twins Discordant for Obesity Modulate Metabolism in Mice." *Science* 341, no. 6150 (September 6, 2013). http://science .sciencemag.org/content/sci/341/6150/1241214.full.pdf.

Chapter 4: Better Gut Health, Less Disease

American Heart Association. "Gut Bacteria Hold Clues to Heart Health." http://news .heart.org/gut-bacteria-hold-clues-to-heart-health/.

Cénit, M. C. et al. "Rapidly Expanding Knowledge on the Role of the Gut Microbiome in Health and Disease." *Biochimica et Biophysica Acta* 1842, no. 10 (October 2014): 1981–1992. http://ac.els-cdn.com/S0925443914001513/1-s2.0 -S0925443914001513-main.pdf?_tid=42be934c-ea48-11e5-8f0f-00000aacb 361&acdnat=1458003358_42eaa4aa81c73ce430a1e54a4a88e5a9.

Centers for Disease Control and Prevention. "Chronic Disease Overview."
http://www.cdc.gov/chronicdisease/overview/index.htm?s_cid=ostltsdyk
_govd_203.

Centers for Disease Control and Prevention. "Epidemiology of the IBD." http://www.cdc
.gov/ibd/ibd-epidemiology.htm.

Centers for Disease Control and Prevention. "Trends in Allergic Conditions Among Children: United States, 1997–2011." http://www.cdc.gov/nchs/products/databriefs
/db121.htm.

Centers for Disease Control and Prevention. "What Is Inflammatory Bowel Disease?"
https://www.cdc.gov/ibd/what-is-ibd.htm.

Deehan, E. C., and J. Walter. "The Fibre Gap and the Disappearing Gut Microbiome:
Implications for Human Nutrition." *Trends in Endocrinology & Metabolism* 27, no. 5 (2016):
239–242. http://www.cell.com/trends/endocrinology-metabolism/fulltext/S1043
-2760(16)00035-7.

Khanna, S., and P. K. Tosh. "A Clinician's Primer on the Role of the Microbiome in Human
Health and Disease." *Mayo Clinic Proceedings* 89, no. 1 (January 2014): 107–114.
http://www.mayoclinicproceedings.org/article/S0025-6196%2813%2900886-0
/pdf.

Kitai, T., J. Kirsop, and W. H. Tang. "Exploring the Microbiome in Heart Failure." *Current
Heart Failure Reports* 13, no. 2 (April 2016): 103–9. http://link.springer.com/article
/10.1007%2Fs11897-016-0285-9.

Montassier, E. et al. "Chemotherapy-Driven Dysbiosis in the Intestinal Microbiome."
Alimentary Pharmacology and Therapeutics 42 (2015): 515–528. http://www.drperl
mutter.com/wp-content/uploads/2015/09/Montassier_et_al-2015-Alimentary
_Pharmacology__Therapeutics.pdf.

National Institute of Diabetes and Digestive and Kidney Diseases. "Definition and Facts
for Irritable Bowel Syndrome." https://www.niddk.nih.gov/health-information
/health-topics/digestive-diseases/irritable-bowel-syndrome/Pages/definition-facts
.aspx.

Shreiner, A. B., J. Y. Kao, and V. B. Young. "The Gut Microbiome in Health and in
Disease." *Current Opinions in Gastroenterology* 31, no. 1 (January 2015): 69–75.
http://www.ncbi.nlm.nih.gov/pmc/articles/PMC4290017/.

Yamamoto, M. L. et al. "Intestinal Bacteria Modify Lymphoma Incidence and Latency by
Affecting Systemic Inflammatory State, Oxidative Stress, and Leukocyte Genotoxicity."
Journal of Cancer Research 73, no. 14 (July 2013). http://cancerres.aacrjournals
.org/content/73/14/4222.abstract.

Chapter 5: Start Repairing Gut Damage TODAY

David, Lawrence A. et al. "Diet Rapidly and Reproducibly Alters the Human Gut Microbiome." *Nature* 505 (January 23, 2014): 559–563. http://www.ncbi.nlm.nih.gov/pmc/articles/PMC3957428/.

Deehan, E. C., and J. Walter. "The Fibre Gap and the Disappearing Gut Microbiome: Implications for Human Nutrition." *Trends in Endocrinology & Metabolism* 27, no. 5 (2016): 239–242. http://www.cell.com/trends/endocrinology-metabolism/fulltext/S1043-2760(16)00035-7.

Chapter 6: Feed Your Buddies the Food They Love Best

Centers for Disease Control and Prevention. "Morbidity and Mortality Weekly Report." http://www.cdc.gov/mmwr/preview/mmwrhtml/mm6426a1.htm.

Harvard School of Public Health. "The Nutrition Source: Fibre." https://www.hsph.harvard.edu/nutritionsource/carbohydrates/fibre/.

Mayo Clinic. "Chart of High-Fibre Foods." http://www.mayoclinic.org/healthy-lifestyle/nutrition-and-healthy-eating/in-depth/high-fibre-foods/art-20050948.

National Academies of Sciences, Engineering, and Medicine. "Dietary Reference Intakes for Energy, Carbohydrate, Fibre, Fat, Fatty Acids, Cholesterol, Protein, and Amino Acids." http://nationalacademies.org/hmd/reports/2002/dietary-reference-intakes-for-energy-carbohydrate-fibre-fat-fatty-acids-cholesterol-protein-and-amino-acids.aspx.

Palmer, S. "The Top Fibre-Rich Foods List." *Today's Dietitian*, July 2008. http://www.todaysdietitian.com/newarchives/063008p28.shtml.

USDA Nutrition Insight 36. "The Food Supply and Dietary Fibre: Its Availability and Effect on Health." http://www.cnpp.usda.gov/sites/default/files/nutrition_insights_uploads/Insight36.pdf.

Yunsheng, Ma et al. "Single-Component vs. Multicomponent Dietary Goals for the Metabolic Syndrome: A Randomized Trial." *Annals of Internal Medicine* 162, no. 4 (February 17, 2015): 248–257. http://annals.org/article.aspx?articleid=2118594.

Chapter 7: Fill Your Belly with Prebiotic Superstars

Harvard T.H. Chan School of Public Health. "Vegetables and Fruits." https://www.hsph.harvard.edu/nutritionsource/what-should-you-eat/vegetables-and-fruits/.

Chapter 8: Pick Plenty of Plant Protein

Bao, Y. et al. "Association of Nut Consumption with Total and Cause-Specific Mortality." *New England Journal of Medicine* 369 (November 21, 2013): 2001–2011. http://www.nejm.org/doi/full/10.1056/NEJMoa1307352.

Harvard T.H. Chan School of Public Health. "Eating Nuts Linked to a Longer, Healthier Life." http://www.health.harvard.edu/blog/eating-nuts-linked-to-healthier-longer-life-201311206893.

Health and Medicine Division of the National Academies of Sciences, Engineering, and Medicine. "Dietary Reference Intakes: Macronutrients." http://www.nationalacademies.org/hmd/~/media/Files/Activity%20Files/Nutrition/DRIs/DRI_Macronutrients.pdf?la=en.

Pan, A. et al. "Red Meat Consumption and Mortality: Results from Two Prospective Cohort Studies." *Archives of Internal Medicine* 172 (April 9, 2012): 555–63. http://archinte.jamanetwork.com/article.aspx?articleid=1134845.

Pan, An et al. "Red Meat Consumption and Risk of Type-2 Diabetes: 3 Cohorts of U.S. Adults and an Updated Meta-Analysis." *American Journal of Clinical Nutrition* 94, no. 4 (October 2011): 1088–96. http://ajcn.nutrition.org/content/94/4/1088.full.

Song, M. et al. "Association of Animal and Plant Protein Intake with All-Cause and Cause-Specific Mortality." *JAMA Internal Medicine* (August 1, 2016). http://archinte.jamanetwork.com/article.aspx?articleid=2540540.

World Health Organization. "Q&A on the Carcinogenicity of the Consumption of Red Meat and Processed Meat." http://www.who.int/features/qa/cancer-red-meat/en/.

Chapter 9: Don't Give Up on Grains!

Aune, D. et al. "Whole Grain Consumption and Risk of Cardiovascular Disease, Cancer, and All-Cause Specific Mortality: Systematic Review and Dose-Response Meta-Analysis of Prospective Studies." *BMJ* 353 (May 2016). http://www.bmj.com/content/353/bmj.i2716.

Foerster, J. et al. "The Influence of Whole Grain Products and Red Meat on Intestinal Microbiota Composition in Normal Weight Adults: A Randomized Crossover Intervention Trial." *PLoS One* (October 9, 2014). http://journals.plos.org/plosone/article?id=10.1371/journal.pone.0109606.

Food for Life. "7 Sprouted Grains Bread." http://www.foodforlife.com/product/breads/7-sprouted-grains-bread and www.foodforlife.com/product/breads/ezekiel-49-sprouted-whole-grain-bread.

Liu, S. et al. "Whole-Grain Consumption and Risk of Coronary Heart Disease: Results from the Nurses' Health Study." *American Journal of Clinical Nutrition 70 (1999):* *412–9.* http://ajcn.nutrition.org/content/70/3/412.long.

Martinez, I. et al. "Gut Microbiome Composition Is Linked to Whole Grain-Induced Immunological Improvements." *ISME Journal* 7, no. 2 (February 2013): 269–80. http://www.nature.com/ismej/journal/v7/n2/full/ismej2012104a.html.

Oldways Whole Grains Council. "What Is a Whole Grain?" http://wholegrainscouncil .org/whole-grains-101/what-is-a-whole-grain.

Chapter 10: Get Your Buddies to Go

Bubbie's. http://bubbies.com/.

Elli, M. et al. "Survival of Yogurt Bacteria in the Human Gut." *Applied and Environmental Microbiology* 72, no. 7 (July 2006): 5113–5117. http://www.ncbi.nlm.nih.gov/pmc /articles/PMC1489325/.

Siggi's Dairy. http://siggisdairy.com/.

Sunja's Kimchi. "About Kimchi." http://sunjaskimchi.com/about-kimchi/.

Wallaby Organic. http://www.wallabyyogurt.com/.

Chapter 11: Ban Bacteria Bullies in Food

American Medical Association. "AMA Continues Efforts to Combat Antibiotic Resistance." http://www.ama-assn.org/ama/pub/news/news/2015/2015-11-16-combat -antibiotic-resistance.page.

Consumers Union. "The Overuse of Antibiotics in Farm Animals Threatens Public Health." http://consumersunion.org/news/the-overuse-of-antibiotics-in-food -animals-threatens-public-health-2/.

Environmental Working Group. "Clean 15." https://www.ewg.org/foodnews/clean _fifteen_list.php.

Environmental Working Group. "Dirty Dozen." https://www.ewg.org/foodnews/dirty _dozen_list.php.

Chapter 12: Avoid Unnecessary Antibiotics

Alharbi, Sulaiman Ali et al. "What If Fleming Had Not Discovered Penicillin?" *Saudi Journal of Biological Sciences* 21, no. 4 (September 2014): 289–293. http://www .sciencedirect.com/science/article/pii/S1319562X14000023.

Centers for Disease Control and Prevention. "1 in 3 Antibiotic Prescriptions Unnecessary." http://www.cdc.gov/media/releases/2016/p0503-unnecessary-prescriptions.html.

Centers for Disease Control and Prevention. "Ear Infections." http://www.cdc.gov
/getsmart/community/for-patients/common-illnesses/ear-infection.html.

Centers for Disease Control and Prevention. "Measuring Outpatient Antibiotic
Prescribing." http://www.cdc.gov/getsmart/community/programmes-measurement
/measuring-antibiotic-prescribing.html.

Langdon, Amy, Nathan Crook, and Gautam Dantas. "The Effects of Antibiotics on the
Microbiome Throughout Development and Alternative Approaches for Therapeutic
Modulation." *Genome Medicine* 8 (2016). https://genomemedicine.biomedcentral
.com/articles/10.1186/s13073-016-0294-z.

Chapter 13: Strengthen Your Buddies with Exercise

American Heart Association. "Walk, Don't Run, Your Way to a Healthy Heart."
http://www.heart.org/HEARTORG/HealthyLiving/PhysicalActivity/Walking
/Walk-Dont-Run-Your-Way-to-a-Healthy-Heart_UCM_452926_Article.jsp#
.V6To4jXlZQ0.

Cerda, B. "Gut Microbiota Modification: Another Piece of the Puzzle in the Benefits of
Physical Exercise in Health." *Frontiers in Physiology* 7 (February 2016): article 51.
http://www.ncbi.nlm.nih.gov/pmc/articles/PMC4757670/.

Cleveland Clinic. "What Does Moderate Exercise Mean, Anyway?" https://health
.clevelandclinic.org/2015/04/what-does-moderate-exercise-mean-anyway/.

Hamer, Mark, Kim L. Lavoie, and Simon L. Bacon. "Taking Up Physical Activity Later in
Life and Healthy Aging: The English Longitudinal Study of Aging." *British Journal of
Sports Medicine* 48, no. 3 (February 2014): 239–243. http://bjsm.bmj.com/content
/early/2013/10/28/bjsports-2013-092993.abstract.

Chapter 14: Consider Probiotic Supplements

Agency for Healthcare Research and Quality. "Safety of Probiotics Used to Reduce Risk
and Prevent or Treat Disease." http://www.ahrq.gov/research/findings/evidence
-based-reports/probiotsum.html.

Islam, Saif Ul. "Clinical Uses of Probiotics." *Medicine* (Baltimore) 95, no. 5 (February
2016): e2658. http://www.ncbi.nlm.nih.gov/pmc/articles/PMC4748908/.

National Institute of Diabetes and Digestive and Kidney Diseases. "Definition and Facts
for Irritable Bowel Syndrome." http://www.niddk.nih.gov/health-information
/health-topics/digestive-diseases/irritable-bowel-syndrome/Pages/definition
-facts.aspx.

National Institutes of Health, National Center for Complementary and Integrative Health. "Probiotics." https://nccih.nih.gov/health/probiotics/introduction.htm.

National Institutes of Health, National Center for Complementary and Integrative Health. "Five Things to Know About Probiotics." https://nccih.nih.gov/health/tips /probiotics.

Nazareth, S. et al. "Widespread Contamination of Probiotics with Gluten, Detected by Liquid Chromatography-Mass Spectrometry." *Gastroenterology* 148, no. 4 (April 2015): supplement 1, S-28. http://www.gastrojournal.org/article /S0016-5085(15)30097-4/abstract.

Schneiderhan, J., T. Master-Hunter, and A. Locke. "Targeting Gut Flora to Treat and Prevent Disease." *Journal of Family Practice* 65, no. 1 (January 2016): 34–38. http://www.jfponline.com/specialty-focus/nutrition/article/targeting-gut-flora -to-treat-and-prevent-disease/fae361971eb9601f1c2a720016f976c1.html.

US Food and Drug Administration. "Dietary Supplements Containing Live Bacteria or Yeast in Immunocompromised Persons: Warning—Risk of Invasive Fungal Disease." http://www.fda.gov/Safety/MedWatch/SafetyInformation/SafetyAlertsforHuman MedicalProducts/ucm426331.htm.

Chapter 15: Protect and Support Your Family's Buddies

Bluestein, Jan, and Jianmeng Liu. "Time to Consider the Risks of Cesarean Delivery for Long-Term Child Health." *British Medical Journal* (June 2015). http://www.bmj.com /content/350/bmj.h2410.

Callaway, Ewen. "Scientists Swab C-Section Babies with Mothers' Microbes." Nature.com, http://www.nature.com/news/scientists-swab-c-section-babies-with-mothers -microbes-1.19275.

Centers for Disease Control and Prevention. "Births, Method of Delivery." http://www.cdc.gov/nchs/fastats/delivery.htm.

Centers for Disease Control and Prevention. "Breastfeeding Report Card." https://www.cdc.gov/breastfeeding/pdf/2014breastfeedingreportcard.pdf.

Dominguez-Bello, Maria et al. "Partial Restoration of the Microbiota of Cesarean- Born Infants via Vaginal Microbial Transfer." *Nature Medicine* 22, no. 3 (March 2016): 250–253. http://www.nature.com/articles/nm.4039.epdf?referrer _access_token=clDFvKNFzpliY5_yw2DcA9RgN0jAjWel9jnR3ZoTv0N52P -sU0SaylioNKJaxyGdBjwIdD_rbzx5nhtex-QKrHAO2un_jL6-UpeN7Qo0 QDNxFa_t1l2-A2mH6Q87ASAkyxKGss-Jh6rh75XTAypd4WFa5rZhjpbRdb G1btRwJZRe1g2ulmrAgSSAu4M_-xnYeMRjFb_I_olhhjoV0pyZSeWJ1uD2qbuB _Dbd02zqk8k%3D&tracking_referrer=www.nature.com.

Haelle, Tara. "Your Biggest C-Section Risk May Be Your Hospital." *Consumer Reports,* April 2016. http://www.consumerreports.org/doctors-hospitals/your-biggest-c -section-risk-may-be-your-hospital/.

Khanna, S., and P. K. Tosh. "A Clinician's Primer on the Role of the Microbiome in Human Health and Disease." *Mayo Clinic Proceedings* 89, no. 1 (January 2014): 107–114. http://www.mayoclinicproceedings.org/article/S0025-6196%2813%2900886-0 /pdf.

Office of Women's Health, US Department of Health and Human Services. "Breastfeeding." http://www.womenshealth.gov/breastfeeding/breastfeeding-benefits.html.

Thomas, Dan W. et al. "Clinical Report—Probiotics and Prebiotics in Pediatrics." *Pediatrics* 126, no. 6 (December 2010): 1217–1231. http://pediatrics.aappublications.org /content/pediatrics/early/2010/11/29/peds.2010-2548.full.pdf.

Chapter 16: Get Dirtier

Bates, Karl L. "A Little Dirt Won't Hurt." *Duke,* Summer 2016. http://dukemagazine.duke .edu/article/a-little-dirt-wont-hurt.

Fishbein, R. "Licking Subway Poles Probably Fine, Says Expert." *Gothamist,* February 5, 2015. http://gothamist.com/2015/02/05/quit_cryin_mama_loves_u.php

Holbreich, M. et al. "Amish Children Living in Northern Indiana Have a Very Low Prevalence of Allergic Sensitization." *Journal of Allergy and Clinical Immunology* 129, no. 6 (June 2012): 1671–1673. http://www.jacionline.org/article/S0091 -6749(12)00519-2/abstract.

Stein, M. M. et al. "Innate Immunity and Asthma Risk in Amish and Hutterite Farm Children." *New England Journal of Medicine* 375, no. 5 (August 4, 2016): 411–421. http://www.nejm.org/doi/full/10.1056/NEJMoa1508749.

Recipe Guide Index

About the Author

Dr. Travis Stork is an Emmy®-nominated host of the award-winning talk show *The Doctors*, and a board-certified emergency medicine physician. He graduated magna cum laude from Duke University as a member of Phi Beta Kappa and earned his M.D. with honors from the University of Virginia, being elected into the prestigious honor society of Alpha Omega Alpha for outstanding academic achievement.

Based on his experiences as an ER physician, Dr. Stork is passionate about teaching people simple methods to prevent illness before it happens, with the goal of maximizing time spent enjoying life while minimizing time spent as a "patient."

Dr. Stork is a *New York Times* #1 bestselling author of *The Doctor's Diet*, *The Doctor's Diet Cookbook*, *The Lean Belly Prescription*, and *The Doctor Is In: A 7-Step Prescription for Optimal Wellness*.

An avid outdoorsman, Dr. Stork is a devotee of mountain and road biking, white-water kayaking and hiking with his loyal dog of nearly seventeen years, Nala.